JAIME BRENKUS'
Get Lean
in 15

15 WAYS IN 15 DAYS TO
SHAPE UP AND SLIM DOWN...
FAST!

GET LEAN IN 15

PUBLISHED by FIT 15, LLC

For information:
Fit 15, LLC
2148 Pelham Parkway
Building 300
Pelham, AL 35124
www.fit15.com

ISBN 13: 978-0-9793015-2-0
ISBN 10: 0-9793015-2-1

Printed in the United States of America

Acknowledgments

This book is dedicated to my lovely daughter Lauren, who is my inspiration and to my terrific, understanding wife Teri –who has mastered the art of patience and has to put up with me on a daily basis. Lauren would not forgive me if I left out our other family member -her puppy, Princess. Special thanks to my parents for always being my greatest fans and always being there for me. They have also taught me strong work ethics and the value of perseverance.

A heartfelt thanks goes to the Fit 15 team - I couldn't have asked for better partners.

Finally, I want to thank all of you, who entrusted and believed in me and, for allowing me to help you gain self-empowerment from a new lifestyle…. and a new wardrobe!

Ingredients

Introduction

"SUCCESS IN LIFE IS NOT ABOUT A MATTER OF INCHES OR POUNDS; RATHER, SUCCESS IS WHEN YOU START TAKING STEPS TOWARDS A REACHABLE GOAL"
- Anonymous

The first thing you did this morning was walk to the bathroom and considered getting on the scale. Depending if it's a "fat' or "skinny" day, you might take a look at yourself (fully naked if you're feeling really optimistic that day) in the mirror on the way to the bathroom.

In a smoky, hazy cloud three numbers appear on the scale and your whole day will be decided on what these numbers say. Your body is something you constantly think about throughout the day, and depending on the size, (or your perception of your size) it affects your mood and outlook on life. Those three numbers on the scale will dictate whether or not you should wear your "fat jeans" or your "fit jeans" today. Be honest, isn't it true that if the scale does show your ideal weight, you still wish you had better defined muscles in the legs…or could smooth out your cellulite… or had a tighter waistline.

Let's face it, very few of us are ever completely satisfied with our bodies. This fact brings us to the infamous, tormenting, no results weight loss solution…the DIET.

We all remember the "fat periods" in our lives when we really packed on the pounds, and then through some excruciating diet program we took the weight off, only to have it creep back, or in some cases, to return with a vengeance as soon as we went off the diet program. Then no matter what type of success we had achieved, in terms of pure weight loss, or how good we looked, we never thought we looked good enough.

Am I right so far?

Either our chest was too small or our saddlebags stuck out too much or there was still a visible paunch in the belly or … you name the other flawed parts. The point is that we are always in a constant struggle to achieve the "perfect body." (by the way….no one's perfect)

Why do we spend so much of our time and energy in search of the Holy Body Grail? We try every type of diet, join health clubs, count fat grams, exercise to videos, choke down diet pills and devour prepackaged foods that taste like cardboard; only to be disappointed with the lack of results. Then if we do lose some weight, we systematically gain it back…and then some. In some cases, when we do find an exercise plan that works, we most likely will lack the motivation to follow it for any given period of time. Yet, we continually partake in this DIET cycle.

We need a system that we can do at home and that will fit our busy schedules. We need a program that we can really believe in… not another gimmick. We're tired of getting misled by the fitness/weight loss industry, and all the hipsters and hucksters touting the next "miracle" for weight control. It makes us angry when we think of all the people who have lied or made false promises to us, as well as, taking our money. Where were those people when our programs failed?

The time has come for a real weight management program designed for real people, who have real problems, with real schedules, but who still want real results! I'm going to give you that program. My program will inspire and motivate you in a way that will allow you to finally take **CONTROL OF YOUR LIFESTYLE, YOUR HEALTH, YOUR FIGURE, YOUR ATTRACTIVENESS AND YOUR WELL-BEING ONCE AND FOR ALL!**

Make no mistake, you did *not* fail those diet programs in the past…. they **FAILED YOU!**

The reason why 95 percent of all traditional diets fail is simple. When you go on a diet that is too restrictive, your body believes it is starving, which forces it to actually become more efficient at storing fat by *slowing down* your metabolism, which is not a good thing. If you then abruptly stop this unrealistic eating plan, your metabolism continues to run at a slower and more inefficient pace, which causes you to gain the weight back at an even faster pace. You may even be eating less than you were before you went on the diet. In addition, very low-calorie diets cause you to lose both lean muscle tissue and fat in equal amounts. However, when you eventually gain the weight back, it's all fat and not muscle, causing your metabolism to slow down even more. Now you have extra inches, a less healthy body composition, and no sexy curves or chiseled abs. This is a vicious cycle, a cycle that I am prepared to help you break.

I am going to show you how you never have to "diet" again, if you follow my plan for a healthy lifestyle. My approach to exercise is sensible and painless. You don't have to be a marathon runner or a body builder to see results with my program. By the way, I know that you're busy; however, if you can fit me into your schedule, then together we WILL produce some amazing results. I'll help you to build those sexy muscles that you've been wanting and dreaming about.

My solution isn't difficult. There will be no more crash dieting, fake food, diet pills, or wasting time at weight loss meetings or endless hours at the gym. You'll feel like you're eating your favorite foods and you will **NEVER** feel like you're starving again. You'll also be relieved that you won't have to buy food that's different from the rest of your family.

In order to succeed at your weight management program, everything you eat and every exercise you do must be a pleasurable experience. If you're not having fun and not confident about what you are doing, you'll drop out of your program. It's that simple.

The way to keep motivated is through small **Daily Victories** that are not painful or overwhelming. Instead they are the core of an exciting new lifestyle that you will look forward to.

This program is about long-term R-e-s-u-l-t-s.

I know that if you do not gain results, you'll lose interest, and your program will fail. I know my program works…because I live it everyday. Allow me to help you attain your vision of good health.

I've helped millions of people obtain a slimmer, trimmer, tighter waistline with my 8 Minute Abs exercise videos. Now, I have an exciting, brand new way for you to achieve your dream body…by simply eating the foods you love and fitting in a 15-minute fitness plan every day.

Like most Americans, you've probably tried hundreds of diets, lost some weight and unfortunately gained it back and then some. These diets made you feel like you were incompetent.

We're human, food shouldn't be a punishment. I'm going to show you how to do it the honest way. For instance, you can have a piece of chocolate cake in addition to a healthy diet as long as it's in moderation and just occasionally. So go ahead and have the cake and really enjoy it. It's that simple…and you don't have to beat yourself up over it. Quite frankly, who wants to? Life's too short to be on a "diet' all the time.

The greatest benefit with **GET LEAN IN 15** is that you *don't* have to be perfect. No one is perfect. After the initial 15 days on my plan, if you follow my system just 75 percent of the time …you will succeed on a daily, monthly, yearly basis.

I'm not going to disrupt your lifestyle… I will show you that you can eat the foods you love and crave … and still lose the weight. The best part about my plan is that you can live a lean lifestyle forever. So what do you have to lose? Allow me to be your **PERSONAL WEIGHT LOSS COACH!** I guarantee that this **IS** the best system on the market today. It's as though you have your own Personal Trainer and Dietitian at your side.

GET LEAN IN 15 is only 15 days long and I will show you every day… all the ins and outs on how to eat healthy, get lean, stay lean and give you more energy than you can imagine.

Finally, my program is a systematic solution…that will enable you to see real results within the first few weeks. You *can* lose up to 8 pounds within 15 days. You have nothing to lose…but those inches! Best of all you will do it in a way that you can stick with for life. You not only will get to your goal weight, you will STAY there too!

If you're goal this year, is to get in the **best shape** of your life, or if you need to drop a few pounds before that special event in your life…then put your body in good hands…. you can trust me…I will be with you every step of the way…to ensure your success.

You're very important to me and I have a true **passion** to help you become the best that you can be. I'll help you achieve optimal levels of health and fitness and also give you a strong sense of self-empowerment and self-confidence.

With **GET LEAN IN 15**, you now **own** the **SECRETS** to losing weight and eating healthy for life. **GET LEAN IN 15** is a plan that will continue to show you how you can be a slimmer, trimmer, tighter body and it will give you a lifelong blueprint and the tools for a successful, healthy life.

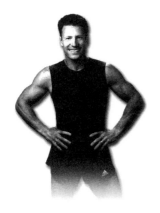

Chapter 1:
Six Steps To Change

We all know how hard it is to change habits – especially when it pertains to food and fitness. I'm going to show you how you can successfully change your habits for the better. I'm also going to change your attitude on how you view food and fitness. First, I need you to think of food for what it really is - a source of fuel for your body. Then, I need you to think of fitness for what it really is – a source of movement for your body.

It's a natural fact of life that everything changes and that nothing stays the same. Change is simply a process. How we react to change, makes all the difference.

There are **6 steps to change** that you will need to understand for your journey towards success. Change is an all-or-nothing proposition. You either do it, or you don't. You can't exercise three times one week, once the next week, take a couple of weeks off, go twice the next week, and so on and expect to reap all the benefits. Or, eat fish once a week and have fried chicken five times and expect to see long-term effects. This isn't reality and usually results in failure. When it comes to your health--jump in with both feet.

Dr. Prochaska, Director of the Cancer Prevention Research Center at the University of Rhode Island, developed a model of six stages of change. Based on Dr. Prochaska's model of change, there are **6 Steps to Change** that people go through regardless if it's to stop smoking, weight loss, alcohol, etc.... It's important to know where you currently fit within these steps of change.

The **Six Steps to Change** are:

* ❋ **Appetite to Lose**
* ❋ **Strong Belief**
* ❋ **Fill up your Plate with Knowledge**
* ❋ **A Plan for Change**
* ❋ **Necessary Ingredients**
* ❋ **Progressing Perfectly**

Step 1. Appetite to Lose

In this instance, appetite means desire. Do you really want to have a lean body? Are you willing to make the necessary effort and commitment to succeed? It's extremely important to want this change to happen so badly that you're willing to face your problems head on and persevere with your goal no matter what obstacles you may encounter. Remember, the hardier your appetite (desire), the greater the likelihood of success. Change for yourself not for someone else. Even if your family and friends want you to do something about your health –it needs to come from within you. You should ask yourself these questions as you begin:

A. **Why do you want to lose weight?**
B. **Are you truly committed?**
C. **Do you have a support system set up?**
D. **Can you accept mistakes without giving up altogether?**

If you answered yes, then move on to the second step.

Step 2. Strong Belief

If you've been on other weight loss plans before and failed –it's OK– remember it wasn't your fault. Your desire to lose may be strong; however, the negative reaction you've had by gaining the weight back may be even stronger. Even if you were not successful in the past, keep thinking you can, you can, and you can! Your attitude will directly affect your weight loss success. That's why it's extremely important that you are convinced that you WILL succeed on this plan. According to Dr. Eliot, "The most important conversations you'll ever have – are with yourself, so watch your language!" I want you to create a vision in your mind of yourself at your ideal goal weight. If you believe this will happen, then it WILL. Start living the lifestyle of your goal weight.

Step 3. Fill up your Plate with Knowledge

This book will be your guide towards your path to change. It's your blueprint for success. Truly understanding weight control and weight management empowers you with the confidence that you'll need in order to succeed. Knowing that you can't or shouldn't lose 10 pounds in a week is important knowledge.

Knowing that the weight didn't come ON overnight, and realizing that it won't come OFF overnight, is important knowledge. The idea of portion control and timely exercise is a proven and effective means towards helping you to reach your goal. When you have the knowledge of eating proper portions, and exercising the right way, then you can make practical and realistic lifestyle choices. All I ask is that you do your best.

Step 4. A Plan for Change

Once you have the desire, belief, and knowledge – you will need a strategy for achieving lasting results. A great plan breaks the process of change into small steps. Follow the plan for 15 days. The smaller steps or **Daily Victories** will make it possible for you to reward and recognize your progression. The GET LEAN IN 15 plan becomes your "home base." It's designed for you to refer back to, even if you fall off track. Take small steps. I like to lead my clients from the grocery aisle -to the kitchen - to the dinner table. By making minor changes without disrupting your lifestyle, is the key to long-term commitment.

Step 5. Necessary Ingredients

You must know that having setbacks are part of the process of change. You will make mistakes and slip-ups will occur. Guess what? – It's OK.

You're going to have days where you want to give up or just binge on food all day long or not do any movement at all. This is a learning lesson. It's another opportunity for you to advance closer to your goal. When you have these setbacks- you MUST realize that this is normal and that you have not failed. How you respond to a setback is extremely important. Just dust yourself off and realize that you have many more days to correct this setback. If you wander off your program for a day or a week – just wander back. It's normal not to be perfect every day on your diet or miss a day working out. These are mistakes that you can correct. Come back stronger and more determined.

Step 6. Progressing Perfectly

Please, you must understand that every time you make a healthy choice, you have progressed. It doesn't matter if you're at your goal weight or not, always reward yourself along the way. Without this positive reinforcement-it's very easy to give up, especially if you've just started and you have to lose a significant amount of weight. Feel good about your accomplishments as you progress toward your goals. Think positive about yourself. Give yourself a pat on the back by going out and buying that new dress or CD you had your eye on - instead of "waiting" until you reach your goal weight. Always keep your motivation and progression moving forward. Feel good about your new, healthy lifestyle- it keeps you marching onward. If you have a lot of weight to lose – focus on the short-term goal of losing a few pounds every week – NOT "I have to lose 100 pounds" – this becomes daunting.

You may be at various levels of commitment in your current lifestyle. Understand these steps of change take time and you may weave in and out of each level until you're ready to move on to the next step. Good Luck and I'll be with you every step of the way.

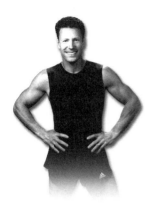

Chapter 2:
Smart Start

Consult your physician before starting this or any other weight management system. If you're a pregnant woman or if you're breastfeeding, you should not embark on a lower calorie diet plan.

The PAR-Q (Physical Activity Readiness Questionnaire) is the gold standard in fitness safety, used by doctors, trainers and health clubs the world over. Usually comprised of 5-7 questions, the PAR-Q can help rule out any underlying health concerns that could worsen with exercise. Please, answer *yes* or *no* to the following questions:

1. Has your doctor ever said that you have a heart condition *and* that you should only do physical activity recommended by a doctor?
2. Do you feel pain in your chest when you do physical activity?
3. In the past month, have you had chest pain when you were not doing physical activity?
4. Do you lose your balance because of dizziness or do you ever lose consciousness?
5. Do you have a bone or joint problem (for example, back, knee, or hip) that could be made worse by a change in your physical activity?
6. Is your doctor currently prescribing drugs for your blood pressure or heart condition?
7. Do you know of any other reason why you should not do physical activity?

If you answer **YES** to any of these questions, then you *must* **check in with your doctor and get cleared for exercise before you start.** I don't need any heroes out there — let's have fun together.

Take your Measurements

Below is a chart that shows you where and how to take your measurements. I'm all about watching your inches drop as opposed to weighing. I believe it's a much better indicator than what the scale is saying.

This is the starting point on your journey to a healthier, more energetic you!

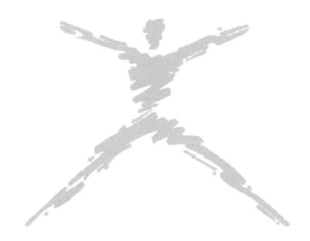

Tape your BEFORE photo here for EXTRA INSPIRATION!

Let's Measure!

Step 1:

I want you to choose a "before" snapshot to paste into the space above, because I want you to remember where you started. Days, weeks, and a few short months from now, you'll be amazed at how far you've come.

Step 2:

You'll want to grab a measuring tape for this next part. Take your measurements and record them in your personal chart. Illustrations and instructions will help you stay consistent when you measure month-to-month. I recommend you measure no more than once a month, but at least once each month.

Step 3:

I've also provided spaces for clothing sizes. While you may not buy new clothes every week, I want you to have space for recording your progress when you do buy something.

You'll be amazed at where you lose inches when you lose weight. Often, watch bands and rings need adjustments. Some people's shoes size even gets smaller.

Below you'll find tips that will help ensure you measure accurately the same way each time you measure your progress. Be sure not to pull the tape too tight! Skin should not "bulge" at the edges of the tape. If you stand in front of a full-length mirror when you measure, then you'll receive more accurate results.

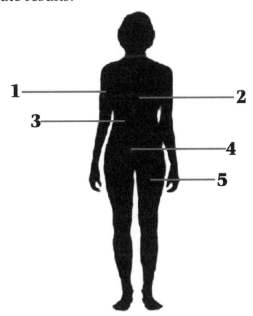

1. **Upper Arm: the widest part of the biceps, only one arm**
2. **Bust/Chest: the widest part, across the nipples**
3. **Waist: midway between the bust/chest and the hips**
4. **Hips: the widest part of the buttock, feet together**
5. **Thigh-single: the widest part of the thigh**

MEASUREMENT/ WEIGHT/ CLOTHING SIZE PROGRESS CHART

MEASUREMENT/WEIGHT/CLOTHING SIZE PROGRESS CHART (FILL IN APPROPRIATE ROW)						
MEASUREMENT	START	WEEK 4	WEEK 8	WEEK 16	WEEK 20	TOTAL LOSS
Upper Arm						
Bust/Chest						
Waist						
Hips						
Thigh - Left						
Thigh - Right						
WEIGHT						
SIZES						
Tops						
Pants						
Skirts						
Dresses						
Jackets/Coats						
Underwear						
Bras						
Pantyhose						
Shoes						
Ring						

Weigh In's

For best results, try to weigh ONLY once a week at the same time and weigh on the SAME scale each week. This is your best indicator for accuracy. As you know, the scale will be deceiving as you become more fit. You will be putting on plenty of muscle tissue—a good thing and losing body fat-also a good thing. However, the scale might look odd if it shows no progress. Your weight will fluctuate from day to day. Resist the urge to weigh yourself on a daily basis, as doing so will discourage you.

Please understand that muscle and fat weigh the same. However, muscle tissue is more compact than fat, and is metabolically active, meaning it requires calories to be maintained. Fat is the opposite. It simply sits there, waiting in case it may need to be used in the future. Fat does not require any calories to be maintained. **Fat is fluffy and bumpy, while muscle is sleek and shapely**. Which would you rather wear?

In fact, two women can weigh the same and, based on their fat-to-muscle ratio, look totally different — either fit and lean, or soft and doughy. So try to focus on more than just the scale! Keep track of your lost inches with the tape measure, too!

Remember, that even if you're gaining muscle weight, you're increasing your fat-burning potential and reshaping your figure at the same time. You're looking great and feeling better — and that's an accomplishment to be proud of!

Instant Body Makeover

Take a picture of yourself and have it "morphed" at a photo shop. Want to see how you look 10, 20, 30 pounds lighter? Have the picture people in the store edit the picture in the image you like, then take home copies of it and hang them everywhere you can see it. Yes--the power of visualization. This really works –try it.

Which BODY TYPE are you?

I need you to be prepared to have realistic goals. It's important to understand that if you have a short, rounded body, there is no way for your body to morph into a taller one. Believe me I know, if that were the case, I'd have worked myself into a 6 foot 4 stature --instead of 5 foot 7.

Physiologists have long classified people according to three body types. Genetics play a role in your physical potential. There are three main body types. You most likely will possess one of these types. Exercise according to your body type and you will see amazing results!!

ENDOMORPHS- round build and gain weight easily -think hourglass figure. Tend to have a higher percentage of body fat –but are strong and have no problem building muscle. Priority: Burn calories to keep body fat down and strength train to increase lean muscle.

MESOMORPHS- typically muscular with a low percentage of body fat and lean physique. Priority: Split routine between Cardio and Strength training.

ECTOMORPHS- usually tall and thin and can eat whatever they want without gaining a pound. Priority: You most likely have a quick metabolism, so you need to emphasize building muscle over burning calories.

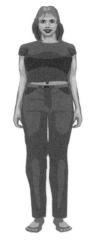 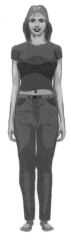 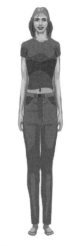

Endomorph   **Mesomorph**   **Ectomorph**

Most people fantasize about reaching a weight that is much lower than they can realistically maintain from a physiological standpoint. You may need to rethink your interpretation of what's realistic. Your goals must match your potentials and limitations. Setting unrealistic goals only invites failure. For example, I was personal training a woman in Florida, Pam, a nurse, about 45 years old. Pam had been overweight for the past 25 years. She came to me and described to me how she longed to be skinny. She said, "I've wanted to be thin all my life- will you help me?" I didn't have a problem with Pam's enthusiasm; however, I did have a problem with Pam's expectations. You see Pam was big-boned with a classic "endomorphic" body. Meaning, she was shorter and rounder. Pam wanted to look like an "ectomorph," someone who is tall and lanky. This was physically impossible. If you're a large framed person, then it is genetically impossible for you to become petite in size.

Genetics play a **huge** role in determining what your realistic expectations are. For example, if neither of your parents is overweight, then there is only a 10 percent chance that you'll be overweight. If one of your parents is overweight, then you are 40 percent more likely to be overweight. Finally, if both of your parents are overweight, then your chances go up to 80 percent.

Therefore, take your body type into consideration and set smaller achievable goals. Remember that thin is not necessarily healthy. I know that if you follow my plan you will become healthy. A great by-product of good health is to become leaner, sexier and fit. Think health first.

MOVING FORWARD

So, how do you measure your progress? Physical indicators of progression towards a healthier body are found in the fat distribution in the waist circumference and waist-hip ration (WHR). Because abdominal obesity has consistently been associated with risk factors for diabetes and heart disease, any reduction in the waist circumference or in the WHR is a positive step towards a healthier body fat distribution, regardless of weight loss.

A better predictor of your weight issue would be to follow the very simple guide of **adult men measuring less than 40 inches around the waist and adult women less than 35.** Although, this is non-scientific, it gives you an idea that if you're over these "safe" numbers, then it's time to start this program!

You've probably heard of "BMI". This is your Body Mass Index. BMI is the standard government measurement used to determine whether or not a person is within a healthy weight range. The BMI chart takes into consideration your weight and height. However, beware that BMI is *not* the best indication of fitness. Someone who is muscular and in shape will have a higher BMI, because of a low-percent body fat, which can be confirmed by using the waist measurement to evaluate fitness. For instance, I'm considered "overweight " by the BMI guidelines, even though I have a low, 8% body fat-I have more muscle tissue.

Determining Your Body Mass Index (BMI)

The table below has already calculated the math and metric conversions. In order to use the table, find the appropriate height in the left-hand column. Then move across the row to the given weight.

BMI (Body Mass Index) Chart

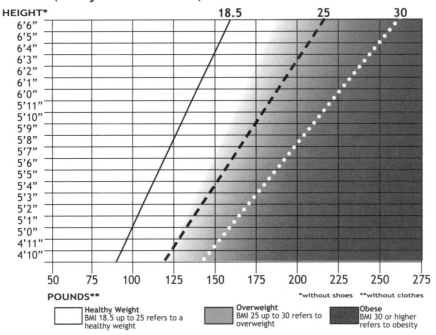

POUNDS**   *without shoes **without clothes

Healthy Weight
BMI 18.5 up to 25 refers to a healthy weight

Overweight
BMI 25 up to 30 refers to overweight

Obese
BMI 30 or higher refers to obesity

Source: Report of the Dietary Guidelines Advisory Committee on the Dietary Guidelines for Americans, 2000, page 3

BMI CHART

BMI measures weight in relation to height. The BMI ranges shown here are for adults. They are not exact ranges of healthy and unhealthy weights. However, they show that health risk increases at high levels of overweight and obesity. Even within the healthy BMI range, weight gain can carry health risks for adults.

Walk the Walk –TALK the TALK

I know while you're exercising, you're always wondering 'how hard should I be doing this activity'? There are a variety of methods for determining exercise intensity levels. Over the years, I have found the most common, simple method is to take the "talk test." While you're working out, if you can hold a normal conversation, then you're doing great. If you can recite the Gettysburg address word for word perfectly –than you need to pick up the pace. However, if you're gasping for air -out of breath…. slow down - you don't have to work that hard. Always, listen to your body-it will generally give you signals that the exercise is too strenuous.

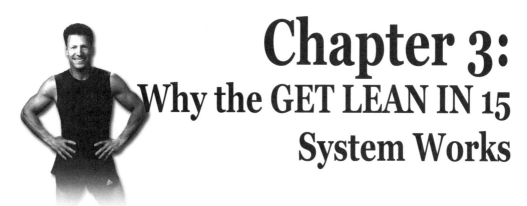

Chapter 3:
Why the GET LEAN IN 15 System Works

It's all here... My system has all the elements and keys to long-term weight loss - although don't be surprised when you see quick results. The keys to long-term weight loss are found in **3 simple steps**. These steps are:

1. **Reducing calories with the foods you love**
2. **Burning calories through movement**
3. **Thinking lean for life-gathering encouragement**

It Only Takes A Few Minutes A Day!

Firming for 15 minutes
Reading 10 minutes
One Daily Victories Action

Why just 15 minutes of exercise?

I've designed your plan based on 15-minute bursts. You'll be combining back-to-back resistance exercises called "Circuit Training." This explosive combination reaps fantastic results. I've been training clients for 20 years utilizing this method—it produces the most desired body in the least amount of time. You'll firm up and tone up, while dropping the pounds and inches. You'll build muscle three days a week with your Circuit Training plan. Then the other three days will be filled with your favorite cardio exercise to burn excess fat. It's that simple.

Exercise ...is the MAGIC Medicine

Fitness is like a piggybank ---it all adds up!!

We all have crazy schedules these days, and the first thing that gets pushed aside in our busy lives is our physical activity. By the time you go to work, make dinner, watch the kids, go shopping, you're busy 25 hours a day –who has time to spend an hour a day in the gym—not many. The great news is that with my program you don't need to.

According to the American College of Sports Medicine, exercise is accumulative –a little here…a little there. You don't have to achieve all your fitness in one session. Small mini workouts will do just fine and in some cases may even be better for you.

Studies have shown, that three 10-minute sessions increase your metabolism three separate times throughout the day as opposed to doing one 30-minute routine. You end up burning more calories. Weight control is about *energy balance*. Nutrition and physical activity are part of the equation. Physical activity has a direct effect on your metabolism, which directly affects your rate of weight loss. If you build one pound of muscle, you'll burn about 50 extra calories per day. Building lean muscle mass will increase your metabolic rate.

Dr. C. Everett Koop, former Surgeon General and the founder of SHAPE UP AMERICA, said that based on what we know now, everyone could find some time to include more activity in their day. The KEY is to think of SMALL WAYS to get the body moving, which will add up to BIG dividends in terms of better health. The opportunity to exercise ALWAYS exists in our lives. It comes down to our choice and what's MOST IMPORTANT at that time. We all have the same 24-hours in our day. It's your choice everyday to either be active or not.

By performing your 15 minutes of exercise six days a week, I know that these 90 minutes (15 X 6 =90) are more beneficial than zero minutes. I'm sure you'll agree. I have high hopes that you'll gradually fit in more minutes as you see quick results. But let's walk before we run.

FAST FITNESS IS A MATTER OF EFFICIENCY

Even a small amount will make a BIG difference. The more unfit the individual ... the more dramatic the difference! So, if you're just starting out, you better get excited because you'll see even more results!! While exercise may seem intimidating at first – you don't have to be a world-class athlete to be physically active. These exercises are well suited for everyone — it doesn't matter if you're age 8 or 88. The workouts will work for you.

WANT POWER

It's very difficult to fit exercise into your daily life. If you miss a day or two – **DO NOT GET DISCOURAGED**. Just keep trying and do your best. Make an appointment with yourself –it's your time –nobody else gets it.

Anything in life worth achieving is worth the work. This isn't about will power. It takes WANT power!! You're going to have to WANT to be firmer, slimmer, healthier and stronger. You'll have to WANT more energy, WANT more vitality and WANT more confidence in your life. Personal pride builds with each bout of exercise completed. Are you ready to start believing it and saying it...I know that you are!!

Why 15 days of menus?

Put the pedal to the metal! I call this my ACCELERATOR phase-the first 15 days on my plan. During this time you will reap the benefits of dropping those inches and weight... fast... while still eating your favorite foods. This is not a conventional DIET –where you have to cut out complete food groups.

As you know, in our society, if we don't see results quickly we get discouraged and usually drop out of any program. WE WANT INSTANT GRATIFICATION. We want it all and we want it now. It's so important to see bodily changes rapidly to keep the progression moving forward.

Kim Tessmer, a Licensed and Registered Dietitian, designed your menus so that you will gain optimum nutrition with a level of calories that will maintain good, positive health, along with helping you shed those unwanted pounds.

I believe that if you're de-conditioned and not in the best of shape, you can safely consume a minimum of 1200 calories and drop unwanted pounds based on pure science. I'm confident that this will give you a negative caloric balance for the day. What is a *negative caloric balance*? When you reach a negative caloric balance, your body is taking in fewer calories than it needs, resulting in you losing weight. If you're in a *positive caloric balance*, then you are consuming more calories then your body is burning off –so the weight keeps coming on.

For all the guys out there, I need you to use the 1400-calorie menus and add additional foods as need be. If you regularly exercise, it's important to add more calories. You always want to be properly "fueled" with food.

I realize on other plans, that you needed to write down every morsel of food in a journal. I'm not going to make you do that. However, if you're really ambitious, keeping a nutrition journal for at least 4-12 weeks is a great idea and an incredible learning experience. But all you really need to get started is one good menu plan-and the menus that Kim and I designed are ideal to guide you on the right path. I've included 15 days of scrumptious meal plans. If you get bored eating the same thing every week, you can create multiple menus, or just exchange foods using your base menu as a template.

Using this method, you really only have to focus on portions when you create your menus. After you've got a handle on calories and portions from this initial discipline of menu planning, then you can estimate portions in the future and get a pretty good (and educated) ballpark figure.

CALORIES COUNT!
According to the American Institute for Cancer Research, 80 percent of people believe that WHAT they eat is more important than HOW

MUCH. In order to lose weight, it is ESSENTIAL to create a *negative caloric balance*, or a calorie deficit. By re-proportioning your food groups according to the GET LEAN IN 15 system, you will have MORE food to eat with FEWER CALORIES left at the end of the day to burn off. It's that simple –you need to eat in order to LOSE!!

Yes, calories do count! Any diet program that tells you, "calories don't count" or you can "eat all you want and still lose weight" is a diet you should avoid. The truth is, that line is a bunch of baloney designed to make a diet program sound easier to follow (anything that sounds like work – such as starting a fitness plan or eating less - tends to scare away potential customers!) Remember that if it sounds too good to be true than it probably is!

The law of calorie balance is an unbreakable law of physics:

Energy in -versus -Energy out

It dictates whether you will gain, lose or maintain your weight.

Good Health isn't about CHANCE. ...It's about CHOICE!!

You are about to embark on an exciting journey. This journey involves learning about your thoughts, feelings and attitudes about food and fitness in a special way. You will learn NEW WAYS to reshape old habits around eating and activity. If you were to ask 500 lean, physically fit people detailed questions about their lifestyles, you would find that they all had something in common:

LEAN PEOPLE LEAD LEAN LIVES!

You would find that these slender, healthy people have similar lifestyle habits that enable them to permanently make weight control a non-issue in their lives. Next to genes, lifestyle habits…eating, shopping, cooking, exercise and even thinking habits ---are the most powerful shapers of the human body.

Starvation is a waste of time and energy. Diets don't change habits!! What matters most is your progress toward weight loss and a healthy body. People take many routes to reach the same goal, you should find the pace at which you feel comfortable and proceed from there.

I'll be giving you one or two new skills to implement every day. Keep in mind that some skills take more time to master than others. It may take some people awhile to learn how to shop effectively, while for others, it may take only a matter of one trip to the grocer. Whatever your rate of change ---please be patient. Changing any habit takes time, determination, discipline, confidence, sacrifice and commitment. Sounds tough-but YOU CAN do it.

I <u>KNOW</u> what works:

Positive attitude
    +Healthy nutrition habits
        +A commitment to exercise
            = Equals a HEALTHY BODY

It is my belief that if your program is to succeed, it can't disrupt your lifestyle. That's why I created your **DAILY VICTORIES QUICK FIX** that will enable you to grasp hold of a new strategy every day for 15 days. By implementing these mini changes daily, you'll be able to adjust to this change without major disruptions in your life. This realistic approach is simple and will focus on doing gentle movements each day, or by choosing a new healthy meal and creating a daily atmosphere of lean thinking.

The process of change happens slowly. By doing a little bit each day-you can build on your successes. By starting with just one or two goals, you can easily ingrain a new habit into your life---- YOU WILL NOT FAIL. Failure is an impossibility when you can have **DAILY VICTORIES. It's self –empowering knowing that you can do it -** without turning your life upside down!!

Don't look backward. But don't look forward, either. Here's why: Each day represents a new 24-hour time clock. By living today — the best you can — the healthy way--this gives you the positive motivation to make tomorrow even better. It's like the principles used at an Alcoholics Anonymous meeting. They don't try to stop drinking forever--they say I will not drink for today.

Every 24 hours represents an opportunity to make it a Daily Victory. Visualize taking all of the steps with this plan and the joy of reaching your goal. Ask yourself "WHAT CAN I DO TODAY TO MAKE THIS GOAL HAPPEN." No goal is ever achieved until it finds its way into your daily thoughts and actions. Then it becomes a part of you.

GET LEAN IN 15 re-programs the way you live your life in regards to health and fitness – so, it's no effort to live this way the rest of your life. If you are striving for, **permanent change** - this system is the one for you. For the past twenty years, I've constantly had people come up and ask me how I stayed so lean? At 46 years old, and still at a healthy, lean 8% body fat, I figured now was the time to write down all my choices and tips to live a lean lifestyle for a lifetime.

Here are my **15 Ways** in **15 Ways** that will enable you to become the lean person that you want to be:

15 WAYS in 15 DAYS

Day 1. All Circuits Go!
Optimum fitness program in the least amount of time!

Day 2. Perfect Portions
Portion control is the key to long-term weight control.

Day 3. Breaking the Label Code
Figuring out nutrition fact labels on food packages.

Day 4. Breakfast is for Weight Loss Champions!
Making right choices in the morning is mandatory.

Day 5. Skim to Slim
Choose fat-free or 1% dairy products --cuts down on unhealthy fats and unwanted calories.

Day 6. Lean Protein
Choosing low-fat or lean proteins at all meals.

Day 7. Winning at Losing
Psychology of how and why you will stick to this plan.

Day 8. Go Green
Include a green vegetable on your plate every day.

Day 9. Drink to Victory
The leanest beverage choices for weight control.

Day 10. Do the Dip
Dipping your fork in salad dressing and other condiments - cuts enormous amounts of fat and calories.

Day 11. Fiber Up
Fiber fills you up…not out.

Day 12. Weigh to Goal
Striving for realistic, positive goals.

Day 13. Empty your Calories
Eliminating one "Empty Calorie " food choice per day will save an enormous amount of calories and help you win.

Day 14. Get Fruity
Eat two pieces or more of fruit daily for proper weight control and good health.

Day 15. One Meal at a Time
Eating your way through any obstacle for weight loss.

It's important to spend a few short minutes a day READING each new DAILY VICTORIES segment. Read each section…apply it to your daily routine…it will change your life!

YOU'VE BEEN WARNED.... YOU MAY NEED A NEW WARDROBE!!!

If you're de-conditioned and out of shape, the ACCELERATOR phase –the first two weeks, may yield some impressive results for you. I've had clients experience a weight loss of up to 8 pounds in the first 15 days. This will not be reached by everyone, but the combination of controlling calories by following our Research and Development designed menus along with an increase in your physical activity, will enable you to burn more calories than you take in; hence, the rapid weight loss. Please understand some of this loss may be attributed to water weight and not fat. The key is to gather the knowledge of what the system brings to you on a daily basis for future healthy weight and inch loss.

In your ENERGIZER phase, the period after a few weeks, you should be able lose 1 to 2 pounds during most weeks. Many weeks, you will not lose anything …and that's OK. Your body reaches natural set points.

A Healthier Weigh

You may be thinking this is all good and well for someone who has a weight issue alone, but what about someone who already has certain dietary restrictions? The $ 30 billion weight loss industry continues to put tremendous emphasis on reaching a healthier weight. That's good since two thirds of the overweight population are more likely to suffer with diabetes, heart disease, high blood pressure, or high cholesterol. The down side for the consumer is that the same people keep losing the same weight. The GET LEAN IN 15 plan will not only help you reach a healthier weight, it will help you *maintain* a healthier weight through the repetition of new behaviors.

If you are one of the 66% who have diabetes, heart disease, high blood pressure, or high cholesterol **AND** you're overweight, I have great news. My menus that I provided for you will work with your dietitian devised meal plan.

The Right Mix

The combination of macronutrients –the calorie providing nutrients– becomes instrumental when trying to lose weight, improve blood cholesterol, improve blood pressure, or improve blood sugar. The fat and protein requires more time to digest so the meal stays with you longer. The sugar from the carbohydrate will also be utilized more slowly in the mix. What does this mean? Your blood sugar will not spike up and down leaving you with a feeling of starvation and crashing (you know the feeling). You will not get hungry between meals!! You will not feel the urge to snack!! Calories will be controlled and the weight will come off.

Remember the emphasis on reaching a "healthier weight?" *Why is it a healthier weight*? **As an overweight person loses just 5-10 pounds, blood sugar, blood pressure, and blood cholesterol will show improvements as well; thus, the new weight is a healthier weight!**

Chapter 4:
15 Days of FITNESS & FOOD
Your Exercise and Menus...............

If you're a beginner, then you need to start off slow and go at your own pace, while you ease yourself into the program. If you haven't worked out for a long time or have never trained before, then don't try to do all the reps at once. Listen to your body. You should *never* be in any pain. My motto is simple: Train don't strain. Starting smart and small helps you to avoid burnout. These mini workouts will condition you for a lifetime of staying fit.

Ladies, I recommend using 3, 5 or 8 pound hand held weights to start. Guys, I recommend using 5, 8 or 10 pound hand held weights to start. If you're more advanced, then you can use heavier weights in the beginning. Please remember to progress at your own ability level. Having proper form is more important than the amount of weight you use. Choose the heaviest weight that allows you to complete all the reps, while taking 3 seconds to complete each repetition…in perfect form. You'll find the exercise photos and explanation in Chapter 7.

The greatest benefit about this workout plan is that you can mix and match the routines. It's like having me there as your Personal Trainer with you at every session. Pick the routines that you enjoy and that meet your body's needs. I advise that once you finish with the prescribed 15 day plan, that you change your routine every 4-6 weeks. This helps to keep you fresh and motivated or join my online membership at www.fit15.com and receive a different routine everyday.

If you feel ambitious and you have the time, then you can advance your exercise plan by repeating the routine over again. This will give you 30 minutes of muscle sculpting.

You will notice with the menus, that the RD and I designed include one daily meal replacement nutritional bar. Put simply, the bars represent a nutritional supplement designed to maximize body fat loss and more importantly, to control your calories.

As you know, I've helped millions of people with their health. And through the years, I have seen the change in our society to focus on **convenience**. Nutritional bars are an easy way to focus on proper balance. It's not always easy to find time to eat. So, if you know you have one of these bars, that will assure you you're getting quality nutrition that's going to help you get fit and stay fit. I eat nutritional bars constantly, either for a healthy snack or when I'm on the run.

There are plenty of bars on the market. I need you to choose smart. The bars should have an ample amount of **calories** and **protein** to fit into our menu plan.

The bar should contain at least **200-250 calories** and a minimum of **15 grams of protein.**

When you eat a diet composed of sufficient amount of protein, you allow your body to burn stored body fat. In other words, the ratio of the carbohydrates, proteins, and fats in your diet determines if you will predominately burn carbohydrates or stored body fat.

There are plenty of imitation bars out there that are "glorified" candy bars. They usually have a high consistency of sugar. These will not fit into this plan.

Just think how good you feel when you eat a more balanced meal, like a chicken breast salad, versus a high-carbohydrate meal like pasta and bread (lacking in protein). Not only are you usually not hungry for many hours after the more balanced meal, you probably don't feel lethargic, irritable, or bloated. Simply put, by adding a little protein and subtracting a few carbohydrates from your diet, you will experience body fat loss, have better energy, and look and feel great.

Look for nutritional bars that are low in saturated fat and **don't contain palm oil or other hydrogenated fats,** or at least contain very small amounts of these fats (less than 2-3 grams or so for every 200 Calories).

Look for bars that are fortified with vitamins and minerals if you are going to replace a meal with a bar. This will help keep your intake of these important substances within a good range and replace the lost nutrients from the foods you are substituting the bars for.

I have found only a few bars on the market that fit this criteria; I've been eating nutritional bars for the past six months, and have found these bars to be extremely nutritious as well as tasty. You can get more information on these bars at www.fit15.com.

Look over the menus in advance and write a grocery list for all the foods. Please substitute accordingly if you don't care for a particular food choice. For example, if you don't like fish, just exchange it for another protein like turkey or chicken.

The following chart will show you different calorie levels based on your individual needs. As you know, the menus are calculated for 1200 calories. However, if you're an active person, you will need more calories. Remember-this is not a starvation plan.

Food is Fuel

Additional Calorie Level Menus

Directions

All additional calorie levels are based on the core menu or the 1200 calorie menu. If your calorie needs exceed 1200 calories, use the following charts to adjust the menu to meet your specific needs.

Use the food list below to adjust your menus accordingly. You can choose to add a new food to your daily menu or to simply increase a portion size of a food already included for that day to get to your target calorie needs.

The core 1200 calorie menu includes ONE nutrition bar. With higher calorie menus you can choose to include one OR two bars in your daily meal plan. If you include two bars you will not need to include as many food group servings each day.

Food Exchange Charts

(Servings indicated should be added to the 1200 calorie menu)

Food groups	1400 cal w/ 1 bar	1600 cal w/ 1 bar	1800 cal w/ 1 bar	2000 cal w/ 1 bar
Meat/protein	1 serving	2 servings	3 servings	3 servings
Starches	1 serving	2 servings	3 servings	4 servings
Fruit	1 serving	1 serving	1 serving	2 servings
Vegetables		1 serving	2 servings	2 servings
Dairy				1 serving
Fats		1 serving	2 servings	2 servings

Food groups	1400 cal w/ 2 bars	1600 cal w/ 2 bars	1800 cal w/ 2 bars	2000 cal w/ 2 bars
Meat/protein			1 serving	1 serving
Starches			1 serving	2 servings
Fruit		1 serving	1 serving	2 servings
Vegetables		1 serving	2 servings	2 servings
Dairy				1 serving
Fats		1 serving	2 servings	2 servings

Food Lists:

(All Items listed are one serving each)

Meats/Protein
1 oz. boneless, skinless chicken breast
1 oz. white meat turkey breast
1 oz. fish (fresh or frozen) cod, flounder, haddock, halibut, trout, lox, tuna (in season), salmon
1/2 cup low-fat cottage cheese
2 egg whites or 1 whole egg
1/2 cup egg substitute
1 oz. lean red meat
1 oz. pork tenderloin
1 oz. low-fat cheese
1/2 cup tofu

Starch
1 slice whole wheat bread
1/2 whole wheat English muffin
1/2 (6") whole wheat pita
1 (6") tortilla
1/2 cup cooked cereal
3/4 cup whole grain ready-to-eat cereal
1/3 cup pasta or brown rice
1/2 cup potato
1 cup squash
1/2 cup yam/sweet potato
3 cups low-fat microwave popcorn
2 rice cakes, (4")
4 slices melba toast
1/4 cup low-fat granola
1/2 cup beans (also add 1 meat/protein serving)
1/2 cup refried beans (also add 1 meat/protein serving)

Fruit

1 small apple
1 small banana
3/4 blueberries
12 cherries
1 cup melon
1/2 grapefruit
17 grapes
1 kiwi
1 small orange or nectarine
1 medium peach
2 small plums

Dairy

1 cup fat free milk / 1% milk
1 cup soy milk, low-fat or fat free
6 oz. low fat or fat free yogurt

Vegetables

1/2 cup cooked vegetables or vegetable juice
1 cup raw vegetables

Fats

1 Tb. avocado
1 tsp. oil (canola, olive, peanut)
6 almonds
1/2 Tb. reduced fat peanut butter
1 Tb. low fat margarine
1 Tb. reduced fat mayonnaise / reduced fat Miracle Whip
2 Tb. reduced fat salad dressing
8 black olives / 10 large green olives
4 halves, walnuts
1 Tb. seeds (sunflower, pumpkin)

DAY 1   DAILY VICTORIES MENU

Breakfast	Lunch	Dinner	Snack
Omelet cooked with cooking spray: *½ c Egg Beaters *½ c mushrooms, green peppers, tomatoes, onions *2 slices whole wheat toast with 1 tsp. jelly *6 oz. low-fat yogurt	*1 nutritional bar *1 ¼ c strawberries	*3 oz. pork chops (grilled or broiled) *1 small sweet potato w/ spray butter *½ c steamed green beans *1 c vegetable side salad w/ 2 Tbsp reduced-fat dressing * 8 black olives *17 grapes	*2 (4-inch) rice cakes *6 oz. low-fat yogurt

DAY 1   LEAN 15 ROUTINE

******You will be performing each exercise 10-15 repetitions (reps). Each repetition should take you 3 seconds to complete.

Exercise	Repetitions	Position
Push Ups	10-15	on floor
Buns Kicks –r	"	"
Buns Kicks -l	"	"
Ab Crunches	"	"
Quad Lifts –r	"	"
Quad Lifts –l	"	"
Bicycles	"	"
Shoulders Press	"	standing
Squats	"	"
One Arm Rows –r	"	w/chair
One Arm Rows –l	"	w/chair
Alternating Lunges	"	

Exercise	Repetitions	Position
Lateral Raises	10-15	
Plie Squats	"	
Bicep Curls	"	
Outer Thigh Lifts r	"	w/chair
Outer Thigh Lifts l	"	w/chair
Triceps Kickbacks -r	"	
Triceps Kickbacks –l	"	
Stationary Lunges –r	"	w/chair
Stationary Lunges –l	"	w/chair
Bicep Curls	"	
Squats	"	
Triceps Press	"	
Buns Press - r	"	on floor
Buns Press -l	"	"
Inner Thigh Lifts - r	"	"
Inner Thigh Lifts –l	"	"
Side Crunches –r	"	"
Side Crunches –l	"	"

Approximate time: 15 minutes

DAY 2 DAILY VICTORIES MENU

Day 2	*¾ c whole grain cereal with *¾ c blueberries & *6 almonds *1 slice whole wheat toast w/ 1 tsp. low-fat margarine *8 oz fat-free milk	*1 nutritional bar *1 peach	*3 oz. salmon (baked or grilled) *1 small baked potato w/ salsa *1 c steamed fresh asparagus *½ c steamed cauliflower *8 oz fat-free milk	*½ c Low-fat cottage cheese *4 melba toast w/ 1 tsp. low-fat margarine

DAY 2 LEAN 15 ROUTINE

CARDIO –15 MINUTES. Your cardio routines will depend on your preferences. You can simply walk outside, march in place at your home, bike inside or out, jog outside or on the treadmill. You can choose to do the elliptical machine, stair climber, rowing or other various cardiovascular pieces of equipment. You can start at **15 minutes** every other day. However, feel free to do as many minutes as your schedule allows. **I just need you to move.**

DAY 3   DAILY VICTORIES MENU

*1 nutritional bar *1 tangerine	*2 slices whole wheat bread *3 oz. white meat turkey *1 tsp mustard *lettuce/tomato slices *1 c vegetable side salad w/ 2 tbsp. reduced-fat dressing	*3 oz. broiled/ grilled skinless chicken breast *2/3 c pasta topped with 1 tsp. olive oil or ¼ c marinara *parmesan cheese (lightly sprinkled) *1 c steamed broccoli *8 oz fat-free milk	*6 oz. low-fat yogurt *1 c raspberries

DAY 3   LEAN 15 ROUTINE

Exercise	Repetitions	Position
Bicycles (abs)	10-15	on floor
Frog Lifts	"	"
Inner Thigh Lifts –r	"	"
Inner Thigh Lifts –l	"	"
Chest Press	"	"
Quad Lifts –r	"	"
Quad Lifts –l	"	"
Reverse Crunches	"	"
Push ups	"	"
Buns Lifts –r	"	"
Buns Lifts-l	"	"
Standing Rows	"	standing
Plie Squats	"	"
Lateral Raises	"	"
Alternating Lunges	"	"
Shoulder Press	"	"
One Leg Squats r	"	w/chair
One Leg Squats –l	"	w/chair
Bicep Curls	"	"
Stationary Lunges –r	"	w/chair

Exercise	Repetitions	Position
Stationary Lunges –l	10-15	w/chair
Triceps Press	"	"
Bicep Curls	"	"
Straight Leg Dead Lifts	"	"
Dips on Chair	"	w/chair
Buns Press –r	"	on floor
Buns Press –l	"	"
Push ups	"	"
Reverse Crunches	"	"
Bicycles (abs)	"	

Approximate time: 15 minutes

DAY 4   DAILY VICTORIES MENU

*1 whole wheat English muffin toasted w/ 1 tbsp. reduced-fat peanut butter *½ grapefruit *8 oz. fat-free milk *½ c low-fat cottage cheese	*1 nutritional bar *1 cup melon	*3 oz skinless chicken breast (grilled/baked) *1 small sweet potato w/ spray butter *1 c steamed green beans *6 slivered almonds *1 small dinner roll w/ 1 tsp. reduced-fat margarine *1 c vegetable side salad w/ 1 tbsp reduced-fat dressing	*6 oz. low-fat yogurt

DAY 4   LEAN 15 ROUTINE

Cardio - 15 minutes

DAY 5   DAILY VICTORIES MENU

* 1 nutritional bar *1 apple	*3 oz. tuna in water w/ 1 tbsp. reduced-fat mayo and 1 tsp. sweet relish *½ whole wheat 6 inch pita *½ c diced onion, tomato, lettuce *6 oz. low-fat yogurt	*3 oz bbq skinless turkey breast *2/3 c brown rice w/ ¼ c black beans and salsa *½ c tomatoes, cucumbers, zucchini tossed in 1 tsp. olive oil *1 c vegetable side salad w/ 1 tbsp. reduced-fat dressing *17 grapes	*1 slice whole wheat toast w/ cinnamon + spray butter *8 oz fat-free milk

Day 5   LEAN 15 ROUTINE

Exercise	Repetitions	Position
Chest Press	10-15	on floor
Overhead Crunches	"	"
Inner Thigh Lifts-r	"	"
Inner Thigh Lifts –l	"	"
Reverse Crunches	"	"
Frog Lifts	"	"
Buns Lifts - r	"	"
Buns Lifts - l	"	"
Chest Flys	"	"
Scrunches	"	"
Standing Rows	"	standing
Standing Buns Press -r	"	w/chair
Standing Buns Press -l	"	w/chair
Shoulder Press	"	"
Squats	"	"
Lateral Raises	"	"
Reverse Lunges - r	"	w/chair
Reverse Lunges -l	"	w/chair

Exercise	Repetitions	Position
Front Raises	10-15	"
Outer Thigh Raises –r	"	w/chair
Outer Thigh Raises –l	"	w/chair
Bicep Curls	"	"
Plie Squats	"	"
Triceps Kickbacks –r	"	"
Triceps Kickbacks-l	"	"
Alternating Lunges	"	"
Concentration Curls -r	"	w/chair
Concentration Curls -l	"	w/chair
Dips on Chair	"	w/chair
Straight Leg Dead Lifts	"	

Approximate time: 15 minutes

DAY 6   DAILY VICTORIES MENU

*¾ c whole-grain cereal w/ 1 small banana *½ c scrambled Egg Beaters *8 oz fat-free milk	*1 nutritional bar *1 peach	*3 oz. grilled halibut *2/3 cup brown rice *1 c steamed fresh asparagus *1 small dinner roll w/1 tsp. reduced-fat margarine *8 oz fat-free milk	*1 c vegetable side salad w/ 1 oz reduced-fat cheese * 2 tbsp reduced-fat dressing *4 black olives

Day 6   LEAN 15 ROUTINE

Cardio - 15 minutes

DAY 7   DAILY VICTORIES MENU

*1 nutritional bar *½ grapefruit	*2 c romaine lettuce *1/3 c cooked pasta *½ c diced tomatoes and cooked zucchini *2 tbsp. reduced-fat Italian dressing *2 (4-inch) rice cakes	*3 oz. taco seasoned lean ground beef on *2 tortilla shells *½ c chopped onions, tomatoes, lettuce *1 oz. reduced-fat shredded cheddar cheese *¼ cup salsa *8 oz fat-free milk	*6 oz. low-fat yogurt *1 small apple

Day 7   **LEAN 15 ROUTINE**

Exercise	Repetitions	Position
Crunches	10-15	on floor
Frog Lifts	"	"
Bicycles	"	"
Quad Lifts –r	"	"
Quad Lifts –l	"	"
Reverse Crunches	"	"
Push ups	"	"
Buns Lifts –r	"	"
Buns Lifts –l	"	"
Inner Thigh Lifts –r	"	"
Inner Thigh Lifts –l	"	"
Overhead Crunches	"	"
Chest Flys	"	"
Lateral Raises	"	standing
Squats	"	"
Shoulder Press	"	"
Alternating Lunges	"	"
One Arm Rows -r	"	"
One Arm Rows -l	"	"
Standing Buns Press –r	"	w/chair

Exercise	Repetitions	Position
Standing Buns Press –l	10-15	w/chair
Front Raises	"	
Stationary Lunges-r	"	w/chair
Stationary Lunges –l	"	w/chair
Bicep Curls	"	
Triceps Kickbacks–r	"	
Triceps Kickbacks –l	"	
One Leg Squats -r	"	w/chair
One Leg Squats -l	"	w/chair
Dips on Chair	"	w/chair

Approximate time: 15 minutes

Day 8   DAILY VICTORIES MENU

*1 nutritional bar *¾ c blueberries	*1/3 c hummus *4 melba toast *6 oz. low-fat yogurt	*3 oz. grilled, skinless chicken breast topped with salsa *1 oz reduced-fat shredded cheddar cheese *2/3 c steamed brown rice mixed with salsa *1 c steamed broccoli *1 c vegetable side salad w/ 2 tbsp reduced-fat dressing *8 oz. fat-free milk	*½ c low-fat cottage cheese *1 ¼ c strawberries

Day 8   LEAN 15 ROUTINE

Cardio - 15 minutes

Day 9   DAILY VICTORIES MENU

*½ c cooked oatmeal w/ ¼ c raisins *1 whole wheat English muffin toasted w/ ½ tbsp. reduced-fat peanut butter *8 oz fat-free milk	*1 nutritional bar *1 small banana	*3 oz. pork tenderloin (baked or grilled) *½ c corn *1 c steamed zucchini *1 c vegetable side salad w/ 2 tbsp reduced-fat dressing	*6 oz. low-fat yogurt *1 hard boiled egg

Day 9   LEAN 15 ROUTINE

Exercise	Repetitions	Position
Standing Rows	10-15	standing
Lateral Raises	"	"
Outer Thigh Lifts –r	"	w/chair
Outer Thigh Lifts –l	"	w/chair
Shoulder Press	"	
Plie Squats	"	
Lateral Raises	"	
Reverse Lunges -r	"	w/chair
Reverse Lunges -l	"	w/chair
Standing Rows	"	
Straight Leg Dead Lifts	"	
Shoulder Press	"	
Outer Thigh Lifts –r	"	w/chair
Outer Thigh Lifts –l	"	w/chair
Standing Rows	"	
Squats	"	
Concentration Curls –r	"	w/chair
Concentration Curls –l	"	w/chair
Dips on Chair	"	w/chair
Alternating Lunges	"	
Bicep Curls	"	
Triceps Press	"	

Exercise	Repetitions	Position
Crunches	10-15	on floor
Quad Lifts –r	"	"
Quad Lifts –l	"	"
Bicycles	"	"
Push ups	"	"
Buns Press –r	"	"
Buns Press-l	"	"
Scrunches	"	"

Approximate time: 15 minutes

Day 10   DAILY VICTORIES MENU

*2 slices whole wheat toast w/ 1 tsp. reduced-fat margarine + cinnamon *6 oz. low-fat yogurt *½ grapefruit	*1 nutritional bar *1 orange	*3 oz boiled shrimp *1 small baked potato + salsa *1 c steamed green beans * 6 slivered almonds, *½ c steamed carrots *8 oz fat-free milk	*ham and cheese sandwich: *½ 6-inch whole wheat pita *2 oz. lean ham *½ c lettuce *diced tomatoes *1 tbsp. reduced-fat mayo

Day 10   LEAN 15 ROUTINE

Cardio - 15 Minutes

Day 11   DAILY VICTORIES MENU

*1 nutritional bar *1 ¼ c strawberries	*3 oz. tuna in water w/ 1 tbsp. reduced-fat mayo *1 tsp. sweet relish *½ whole wheat 6-inch pita *½ c diced onion, tomato, lettuce *1 c baby carrots *8 oz fat-free milk	*spaghetti w/ meatballs: *2/3 c pasta *2 turkey meatballs *½ c marinara sauce *1 small dinner roll *1 tsp. reduced-fat margarine *1 c vegetable side salad w/ 1 tbsp reduced-fat dressing	*6 oz. low-fat yogurt *1 peach

Day 11   LEAN 15 ROUTINE

Exercise	Repetitions	Position
Side Crunches -r	10-15	on floor
Side Crunches-l	"	"
Chest Press	"	"
Scrunches	"	"
Chest Flys	"	"
Inner Thigh Lifts –r	"	"
Inner Thigh Lifts –l	"	"
Chest Press	"	"
Reverse Crunches	"	"
Quad Lifts –r	"	"
Quad Lifts –l	"	"
Standing Rows	"	standing
Reverse Lunges –r	"	w/chair
Reverse Lunges –l	"	w/chair
Shoulder Press	"	
One Leg Squats –r	"	w/chair
One Leg Squats –l	"	w/chair
Lateral Raises		

Exercise	Repetitions	Position
Stationary Lunges –r	10-15	w/chair
Stationary Lunges–l	"	w/chair
Bicep Curls	"	
Straight Leg Dead Lifts	"	
Triceps Kickbacks –r	"	
Triceps Kickbacks –l	"	
Plie Squats	"	
Bicep Curls	"	
Standing Buns Press –r	"	w/chair
Standing Buns Press –l	"	w/chair
Triceps Press		

Approximate time: 15 minutes

Day 12   DAILY VICTORIES MENU

*1 nutritional bar *17 grapes	*seafood salad *2 oz. shrimp *2 c romaine lettuce *1 c tomatoes, cucumbers, zucchini *1/3 c pasta *2 tbsp. reduced-fat dressing *4 melba toast	*3 oz. strip steak *1 small baked potato *1 small ear of corn *1 tbsp. low-fat margarine *½ c steamed broccoli *8 oz fat-free milk	*6 oz. low-fat yogurt *1 apple

Day 12   LEAN 15 ROUTINE

Cardio - 15 Minutes

Day 13   DAILY VICTORIES MENU

*¾ c whole grain cereal w/ ¾ c blueberries *8 oz fat-free milk	*1 nutritional bar *1 small banana	*chicken stir fry: *4 oz. skinless chicken breast *2 tsp olive oil *½ c peppers, onions *½ c broccoli *½ c carrots *2/3 c brown rice *2 tbsp. teriyaki sauce	*6 oz. low-fat yogurt *2 (4-inch) rice cakes *1 hard boiled egg

Day 13   LEAN 15 ROUTINE

Exercise	Repetitions	Position
Scrunches	10-15	on floor
Buns Lifts–r	"	"
Buns Lifts–l	"	"
Push Ups	"	"
Buns Kicks –r	"	"
Buns Kicks –l	"	"
Chest Fly	"	"
Overhead Crunch	"	"
Chest Flys	"	"
Reverse Crunches	"	"
Push Ups	"	"
Buns Press –r	"	"
Buns Press –l	"	"
Shoulder Press	"	standing
Squats	"	"
Lateral Raises	"	"
Alternating Lunges	"	"
One Arm Rows-r	"	w/chair
One Arm Rows –l	"	w/chair
Squats	"	

Exercise	Repetitions	Position
Bicep Curls	10-15"	
Straight Leg Dead Lifts	"	
Triceps Press	"	
Squats	"	
Concentration Curls –r	"	w/chair
Concentration Curls –l	"	w/chair
Outer Thigh Lifts –r	"	w/chair
Outer Thigh Lifts-l	"	w/chair
Triceps Kickbacks –r	"	
Triceps Kickbacks -l	"	

Approximate time: 15 minutes

Day 14   DAILY VICTORIES MENU

*½ c cooked oatmeal w/ ¼ c raisins + cinnamon *½ c scrambled Egg Beaters *6 oz. low-fat yogurt	*1 nutritional bar *1 ¼ c strawberries	*4 oz. grilled salmon *1 c mixed vegetables *small sweet potato w/spray butter *1 c vegetable side salad w/ 2 tbsp reduced-fat dressing	*1/3 c hummus *4 melba toast *8 oz fat-free milk

Day 14   LEAN 15 ROUTINE

Cardio - 15 Minutes

Day 15   DAILY VICTORIES MENU

*1 nutritional bar *1 tangerine	*omelet cooked w/ cooking spray: *½ c Egg Beaters *½ c mushrooms, green peppers, tomatoes, onions *2 slices whole wheat toast w/ 1 tsp. jelly	*3 oz. pork tenderloin (baked or grilled) *1 tbsp. teriyaki sauce *2/3 c pasta w/ 1 tsp olive oil *½ c diced tomatoes + ½ c zucchini *1 c vegetable side salad w/2 tbsp reduced-fat dressing *8 oz fat-free milk	*6 oz low-fat yogurt *1 c raspberries

Day 15   LEAN 15 ROUTINE

Exercise	Repetitions	Position
Squats	10-15	standing
Shoulder Press	"	
Stationary Lunges –r	"	w/chair
Stationary Lunges –l	"	w/chair
Lateral Raises	"	
Plie Squats	"	
Standing Rows	"	
One Leg Squats -r	"	w/chair
One Leg Squats –l	"	w/chair
Shoulder Press	"	
Reverse Crunches	"	on floor
Chest Press	"	"
Quad Lifts –r	"	"
Quad Lifts –l	"	"
Scrunches	"	"
Frog Lifts	"	"

Side Crunches -r	"	"
Side Crunches -l	"	"
Chest Flys	"	"
Crunches	"	"
Standing Buns Press –r	"	w/chair
Standing Buns Press –l	"	w/chair
Bicep Curls	"	
Outer Thigh Lifts –r	"	w/chair
Outer Thigh Lifts –l	"	w/chair
Triceps Press	"	
Standing Buns Press –r	"	w/chair
Standing Buns Press –l	"	w/chair
Bicep Curls	"	
Squats	"	

Approximate time: 15 minutes

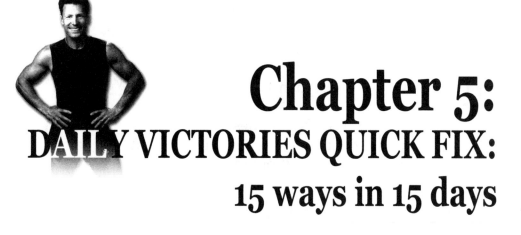

Chapter 5:
DAILY VICTORIES QUICK FIX:
15 ways in 15 days

Day 1
DAILY VICTORIES QUICK FIX: ALL CIRCUITS GO!

"He who has no time for his health today…
will have no health for his time tomorrow"
- Anonymous

I became a personal trainer in Los Angeles in 1986. It was during that time, that I started to take my clients through a series of non-stop movements called Circuit Training. People in the gym thought I was crazy going from one machine to the next, alternating between upper and lower body exercises and various forms of calisthenics. I have always felt this type of routine reaches 99 percent of people's goals; which is lose inches and weight, and firm up at the same time. Circuit Training routines take advantage of non-stop exercises, which allow working muscles to rest in between sets. I've designed your GET LEAN IN 15 workouts to combine both the upper and lower body movements, in each session for maximum results within the least amount of time.

Three days per week, you'll be performing a personalized Circuit Training routine that will tone and tighten your inner thighs, outer thighs and hips in just 15 minutes. These workouts are designed to target every body part and especially some of the trouble spots, such as, your waistline, the back of your arms and your buns. The other three days, you'll be working on your favorite cardio activity. It can be any activity that continues to elevate your heart rate for a minimum of 15 minutes (of course, you can do as many minutes as your schedule allows). **Something** is better than nothing, but **More** is better than something!

Habitually, you spend a few minutes a day brushing your teeth. The same should go for the time you spend on an activity for your body-it becomes a part of your day-without much thought.

MORE MUSCLE = LESS FAT

Muscles not only make your body look sexier; they burn calories at a very high rate.

Burning calories while you sleep!

Get Active ---Lose Weight. The **KEY** is to include resistance training. When you add resistance training to your program at least three times a week, you pack on muscle –and you burn calories **WHILE** you rest. So when you're not working out, your body will burn more calories 24 hours a day, 7 days a week.

This is an important fact to remember. If you gain 1 pound of muscle –you'll burn about 50 extra calories per day. Let's do the math…. If you add 5 pounds of muscle –you'll burn an **EXTRA** 250 calories per day. A body that has 40 pounds of muscle tissue will burn a minimum of 750 to 2000 calories in a 24-hour period –just to stay alive. Now that's how LEAN people stay lean. More importantly, when you put on lean muscle, you increase your resting metabolic rate up to 7.7 percent.

What is all this talk about Metabolism?

Metabolism is the rate at which your body breaks down the nutrients in food to produce energy. Building lean muscle automatically increases your metabolic rate. After the age of 25, most adults lose 3 – 5 percent of their muscle every decade. That's not a pretty sight. That's why we tend to look a little flabbier when we age. We can stave the "sags" as long as we can- by doing resistance training.

Another benefit of a solid resistance program is its effect on our overall appearance and body composition, which can directly influence self-esteem, self-worth, and your level of confidence. Being in better shape, is self-empowering.

For example, a 150-pound woman who has 30 percent body fat- would have 45 pounds of fat weight and 105 pounds of lean body weight (muscle, bones, organs, water, etc.) By beginning an effective strength-training program, she can replace five pounds of fat with five pounds of muscle. She may still weigh 150 pounds; however, she is now 25 percent fat--with 37 pounds of fat weight and 113 pounds of lean body weight. Although her body weight remains the same, her strength, muscle tone, and metabolism have improved, giving her a firmer, fit appearance. YEAH!

One of the biggest mistakes you can make when you start a weight-management program is not to include a strength-training program along with your cardiovascular program. I've always listened to people who said they would like to lose the weight first by doing cardio and THEN they'll start resistance exercises. These are the same people who usually fall off the program, because they don't see RESULTS. **This is a mistake!**

It is unfortunate because when we cut calories without strength exercises, we lose muscle, as well as fat. Many of us choose *not* to do strength training because 1) we mistakenly think it's going to make our body big and bulky, and 2) we don't realize how beneficial and important strength training is in a weight-management program. Whether it is strength, endurance, muscle size, muscle tone or a combination you desire, all are very realistic and obtainable goals with my program.

SPEEDY METABOLISM

Have you ever said to yourself or you've overheard someone say, "I'm gaining this weight because I have a slow metabolism." Let's eliminate that from our dictionary. We will NOT use this phrase again. Studies have shown that only 2 percent of the population has a physical problem enabling them to have a slow metabolism. If you want to REV up your metabolic rate, then get some MUSCLE. People with "fast" metabolism utilize calories more quickly, making it easier to stave off excess pounds.

Plain and simple---Your body's composition is the primary factor for recording the number of calories your body burns at rest. The **more muscle** you have –the **higher** the resting metabolic rate. Lean muscle is similar to the engine in a car. It burns the gas (calories) and provides the power to move. The bigger the engine, the more fuel the car burns.

Since muscle is denser than fat, in a month or so don't be surprised if you put on a pound or two – DON'T WORRY. One pound of muscle takes up less space than one pound of fat. A pound of muscle is like a little chunk of gold, while a pound of fat is like a big fluffy bunch of feathers. Fat takes up more space on your body. Muscle helps you look sexier, trimmer and fitter. Plus, in my program you'll still be eating the foods you love and losing the weight you hate!

Long-term studies indicate that nearly 90 percent of women who dieted and also did a combination of strength training and aerobic conditioning, kept the weight off long-term. Only 30 percent who relied on diet alone keep it off. This fact alone should tell you that the GET LEAN IN 15 approach would work for you.

FOOD FOR THOUGHT: Men have a 10-20 percent higher metabolism than women because they have more muscle. Sorry ladies. This should be apparent as you watch your male friends lose weight more quickly. However, that fact alone should motivate you to do what? .....PUT ON MUSCLE!!!!

After the age of 30, the average woman's metabolic rate decreases at a rate of 2-3 percent per decade – due to INACTIVITY and MUSCLE LOSS. The truth is, that when you're strength training, it's possible to get smaller and heavier at that same time. It is important to make strong, healthy, positive changes, rather, than punishing your body and your spirit through starvation. Your goal is to have a sleek, healthy body of a naturally lean person who can enjoy what they eat. Therefore, you want to avoid at all costs the frail sagging body of a chronic dieter who has to measure every morsel. YUCK!

Women and RESISTANCE

One of the biggest myths is that women will get large, bulky muscles if they lift weights. WRONG! Men have 20-30 times more testosterone than women, and as a result, tend to build more lean body mass than women. Women, will get tight, firm muscles when they lift weights – sounds great doesn't it?

Dieting places a lot of stress on the body and forces the body to lose weight from both fat and muscle. If you do nothing but cardio and never lift weights, you will lose muscle. Many women think that if they just look at a barbell, then they'll immediately begin to look like a big, hairy, grunting bodybuilder. Never happen -- no way, no how. Women just don't have enough testosterone to build large amounts of muscle. Unless you're on steroids, there is nothing to worry about. In fact, the more fat you lose and the more muscle you gain -- the leaner you'll look.

In a study conducted by renowned exercise physiologist, Dr. Wayne Westcott, 72 people followed an exact diet and exercised for 30 minutes three times a week for eight weeks. The 72 people were then divided into two groups. Both groups exercised for 30 minutes -- one group did only aerobic exercise; another group did aerobic exercise and weight machines combination. At the end of eight weeks, the 30 minutes of cardio-only group lost three pounds of fat and a half-pound of muscle. On the other hand, the **combination cardio/weight training group lost 10 pounds of fat and gained two pounds of muscle.** Both groups exercised 30 minutes, but the difference in results was quite dramatic and proves just how effective weight training is.

Weight training has numerous benefits that go beyond just looking better. Resistance training can stave off osteoporosis by increasing your bone mass. By age 70, the average female has lost approximately, 30 percent of her bone mass.

3500 calories ...the magic number

One pound of fat is made up of roughly 3,500 extra calories. This number doesn't change from person to person. That 3500 number's good for me, you and every other person living. In order to lose 1 pound of fat, you need to create a deficit of 3,500 calories. This gives you the basis for the "calories in vs. calories out" type of equation. Simply, you can create a deficit of calories in 2 (or 3) different ways:

Eating fewer calories than you burn each day
Eat anything less than what you use each day consistently, and you'll lose weight. So, if you normally eat 2000 calories per day and all week long you eat 1500 calories per day, you will lose 1 pound (3500 calories) in about a week.

  2000 calories
- 1500
  500 calorie deficit per day X 7 days / week = 3500   or 1 pound fat loss

Exercise More
Keep your caloric intake the same and create your deficit by burning extra calories. So, if you burned 500 calories every day through exercise alone, you will still lose 1 pound in about a week. 500 X 7 =3500.

Combine Both Diet and Exercise
This is the most effective way to lose weight and to keep it off. Let's say you cut your calories by 300 and burn 200 calories with exercise. There is your 500-calorie deficit—with much less deprivation and work. You could speed it up by cutting more calories and exercising more—whatever works best for you. Some people hate to diet; others hate to exercise, so maybe you'll do more or less of either one. Every calorie you burn through activity is GONE FOREVER!!

Learn It!!   Live It!!   Lose It!! .... You'll Love It!!

R U READY?

Studies have shown that seven out of ten people, who start an exercise program, drop out within a few months. **You** are the only person who can take responsibility for the success or failure, of your exercise program. You can't blame anyone or anything for not sticking to your plan. You must be willing to give up a sedentary lifestyle and start describing yourself as an active person.

"If it is going to be ...it is up to me!"

Consistency and persistence are the KEYS to achieving long-term results. If you fall off your program for a few weeks –don't worry. However, if you find yourself constantly making excuses and missing your exercise sessions, you most likely will not succeed. **DO IT !**

Exercise your imagination when it comes to Fitness. It's movement that counts –not fancy machines-nor fancy clothes. **Just keep moving... doing something you enjoy.**

In my 20 years of experience in the health/fitness field, I can honestly say without a shadow of any doubt, that exercise is a **mandatory** component of weight management and physical fitness. The opportunity to exercise ALWAYS exists in our lives. It comes down to our choice and what's MOST IMPORTANT at that time. If you VALUE exercise, then you won't put it in the backseat.

YOU CAN
YOU CAN
YOU CAN

SHAPE UP, SLIM DOWN, GET HEALTHY

A SLIP IS NOT A FALL

Tenacity is one the keys to achieving positive results. Similar to the choices you make with food everyday. Sometimes you'll be pleased with yourself and sometimes you won't. Remember, even a day of missed exercise is a step forward in defining your lifestyle of weight management.

THINK LONG.... THINK WRONG!

Exercise has to be scheduled into your routine and be automatic. Potential interference will strike often. How you respond to these potential interferences is crucial. Be quick to honor your commitment and VALUE yourself.

It's important to explore realistic options while thinking of exercise. I want you to realize that *any* continuous movement will do the job. The activities you choose must be enjoyable, comfortable, convenient and fit within your TIME budget. I need you to focus on movement in general.

BURN BABY BURN

Movement doesn't mean only conventional ways. It just means to get up off the couch and do something.

Ways to burn extra 150 calories	Minutes
Shoveling snow	15
Dancing	20
Scrubbing floors	20
Gardening	30-45
Pushing a stroller	30
Raking leaves	30
Food shopping	40
House cleaning	40
Washing floors	45-60
Washing the car	45-60

I have stayed lean all my life, because I'm always active –always moving. Research has shown that "fidgeting" helps you control your weight. This sounds crazy–but makes the point. If you tap your foot while your sitting at your desk or in front of the TV, then it burns about a half a calorie per minute. If you work a five-day week and burn an extra half-calorie every minute of an eight-hour workday, then you will burn 16 ½ pounds of FAT per year just from twitching. Also, if you want to burn a quick 100 calories, and then tap your foot 9351 times, play the nickel slots at Vegas 234 times, or change 52 diapers. You see, it's not so hard to burn extra calories when you're moving.

MUSCLE MUSIC

I've always found that listening to music is a great diversion while I'm working out. Put on one of your favorite tunes and immediately you want to move with a little vigor. There's a little " pep in your step." Music puts you in the frame of mind that you're doing something that's so valuable to you and yet so much fun. Music can be uplifting. More important, it disassociates you from what you're doing. Before you know it, you'll be finished with your routine. The same goes for putting on the TV while you're on a cardio piece of equipment.

FOOD FOR THOUGHT: More than 75 percent of dieters who are NOT physically active can expect to regain all lost weight within 1-2 years. Exercise is one of the best predictors of successful weight maintenance. This fact should be one of the biggest testimonials towards fitness for you to continue moving.

HEALTHY PRACTICES = HEALTHY BODIES

We don't get a "do-over" in life; therefore, take care of your body. Some things we can control regarding our health. The following facts should motivate you to keep on moving.

- If you're not active, then there is a 3-5 percent reduction in muscle mass each decade after the age of 30, due to a loss of total muscle protein brought on by inactivity and aging

- By age 70, the average female has lost approximately 30 percent of her bone mass. Men at this age have lost approximately 15 percent. Women average a 5 percent decrease per decade after the age of 30

- Your cardiac index declines 20-30 percent from the ages between 30-80

- There is a progressive decline in strength for most muscle groups so that between the ages of 20-70, there is a reduction in overall strength

- Maximum oxygen consumption and endurance show a steady decline in men and women after the age of 20. By age 65, aerobic endurance has decreased by 35 percent

- Your heart's ability to pump blood decreases about 8 percent per decade during adulthood

- For every year you age past 20, your body will lose ½ pound of muscle. For every year you age past 20, you gain ½ -1 pound of fat

- Joint flexibility declines 20-30 percent from the ages of 30-80

- Maximum breathing capacity at age 80 is about 40 percent that of a 30 year old

- Liver and Kidneys lose about 40-50 percent of their function between the ages of 30-70

WOW! Talk about a terrific testimonial to **WHY** you should be physically active and stay in shape. If that's not a wake up call, then I don't know what is. Strive forward with your activity plans on a daily basis and your body will thank you for it later.

7 th INNING STRETCH

A few years ago, I came up with a plan to encourage all Cleveland Indians fans to watch the Indians baseball games and to do short snippets of exercise between innings. The Cleveland Plain Dealer newspaper did a two-page article on this concept.

It was a great way to show everyone that all exercise adds up. For instance, by doing a few sit ups, push ups, squats or lunges during the usual 3 minutes between innings, you could accumulate a great dose of fitness in a very short period. You can also do this for your favorite TV shows. Commercials are approximately 3 minutes every break. It's practical and fun, and you will reap the benefits.

The greatest gift you can give your family is to show them how to stay healthy. As parents, you must lead by example. Exercising together is time well spent.

WALK TO WELLNESS

Despite all the fancy equipment and gadgets we have for exercise these days, the road to fitness can be as easily traveled as putting one foot in front of the other –that's right – by walking. All things considered, walking is the single most practical and effective form of exercise today. No other activity gives you the results of exercise as easily or safely as the simple act of going for a walk or marching in place at home.

Walking is the ideal exercise for those of us with weight issues or those of us who are de-conditioned. It's a natural body movement and doesn't require any special coordination skills. It works our muscles in a consistent, uniform fashion, making it virtually free of the risk of injury.

Even if you're significantly overweight you can walk for weight loss. It may sound like an exhausting proposition; however, studies show that obese individuals need to exert more energy to walk than those of lower weight. But if you begin today, by simply walking to the end of your block, or even just to your mailbox and back, it's a start.

If you currently lead a *very* sedentary lifestyle, then your initial goal should be to walk for 1 minute at a brisk pace on most days of the week. Once you can do this comfortably, increase your distance by adding 5 minutes each day. Walk at a brisk pace, but one in which you can "carry on a conversation."

It's okay to accumulate "mini" walks during the day. For example, you can bet a quick 15-minute walk at lunchtime, or a 15-minute walk before dinner or a 15-minute walk in the evening, all burn those extra calories. Just walk in one direction for 7-10 minutes and then walk back. It's that simple.

Make physical activity a regular part of the day

Don't try to be perfect on your exercise program. There will be days that you just can't do any formal program. That's OK –just keep moving. I have always found that if you schedule a regular time to exercise –you're more likely to stick with the plan. It doesn't matter what time of the day you plan for exercise. However, I have found that morning time usually works the best, because as the day moves along, there become more obstacles that can get in the way.

If you do drop out of your exercise plan, then evaluate the reason why you stopped. Let's make adjustments to prevent future dropouts. Whatever you do, please recommit to a new plan. Make an appointment with yourself. You normally wouldn't cancel a Doctor's appointment would you? So why cancel your own exercise schedule? Put your exercise routine in your day planner. I know that you have something that shows you your schedule. You're worth it –keep it and schedule your activities around it.

I'm only asking for 15 minutes. That's 1/96 of your day. You owe it to yourself for that "ME" time. You deserve it!

See yourself as an active person. Don't let self-image hold you back. Many of us think were too old, too overweight, too tired, not healthy enough to exercise, etc.... These are just excuses. Get out there and move around! Exercise will make you stronger, improve your appearance and give you self-confidence.

Choose activities that you enjoy and that you can do regularly. Fitting activity into a daily routine can be easy, such as, taking a brisk 15-minute walk to and from the parking lot, bus stop, or subway station. Join an exercise class – you get the idea.

More ways to increase physical activity

When I'm on the road, I make an attempt to venture around the city -this gives me a real "feel" for that city and gives me a great way to build an appetite. The hotel four walls get too confining and you could be in your own hometown and watch the four walls. Get out and move about the town.

As you know, these days you need to get to the airport a few hours before your flight. While you're waiting –don't just sit there and read (you can do that on the plane) get up and start walking. This is a great way to expend calories and to relieve the tension that you have about flying. Pacing around the airport while waiting for your flight uses three times the calories that sitting still and staring at your fellow traveler does. I'd advise the same prescription if you're waiting at a Doctor's office.

I always keep a pair of running shoes in my car. Be prepared for any activity by wearing walking shoes or at least comfortable shoes you can walk in. Ladies, I don't know how anyone can walk in high heels. I know when your feet hurt; the last thing you want to do is move more. So, if you bring another pair of shoes with you, then I believe that you stand a good chance at burning more calories during the work hours.

If you go to a ballgame, go for a walk at halftime. At the very least, get up and stretch and move around.

Some more tips on how to burn calories

At home:
- Push the baby in a stroller. I always say- Start em' young

- Get the whole family involved — enjoy an afternoon bike ride with your kids. This is a great bonding time –very positive time spent

- Walk up and down the soccer or softball field sidelines while watching the kids play. 'Kill two birds with one stone'-get fit and be proud of your kids

- Walk up the stairs at least a few times per day. Take two steps at a time to work those buns!

- Walk the dog—don't just watch the dog walk. Our dog looks forward to this and it's a fun way to stay active

- Clean the house or wash the car. Don't forget to provide some extra "elbow grease" when cleaning

- Mow the lawn with a push mower. Give it a try –While I was a homeowner in Florida, I used to run behind an old push mower –what a workout!

- Plant and care for a vegetable or flower garden. I guarantee you'll be doing plenty of squatting motions to weed those roses

- Play with the kids — tumble in the leaves, build a snowman, splash in a puddle, or dance to your favorite music. Be a kid again –let loose and have fun –it's invigorating

- Stop using the drive-thru at the bank, dry cleaner, etc… Park your car, get out and do your errand. We're all guilty of this-including me. However, once you start getting in the habit of parking the car and moving, it makes you feel better about yourself

- Join a walking group in the neighborhood or at the local shopping mall. In my neighborhood, there are a few women who walk every night in the summer…..their jaws get quite a workout too

At work:
- Use the furthest restroom or wastebasket. You may think this is trivial, but every little bit counts

- Get off the bus or subway one stop early and walk the rest of the way

- Replace a coffee or smoke break with a brisk 10-minute walk. Ask a friend to go with you. If you add up all the time that you take breaks hanging out with co-workers - just think of the fitness that you could accumulate

- Get out of your seat at least a few times during the hour and stand up to talk. I make it a point to stand during my conference calls or if I read emails

- Take part in an exercise program at work or at a nearby gym. If this is an option, then it would eliminate driving or any excuse for lack of time

- Join the office softball or bowling team. This not only builds muscles–it builds friendships

- Have a question for a fellow employee -then walk to their desk instead of calling them on the phone or emailing them. Do you want to lose your bottom? Get up out of your seat

Visiting Friends or Relatives:
- Don't just plop yourself down and expect to be waited upon - get up and help. Take their pet out for a walk. Wash the dishes and offer to help clean up

- Before anyone gets up in the morning –go for a walk. Ah, the break of dawn. I promise you when that sun splashes your face in the morning–you will feel rejuvenated immediately

- Take the kid's for a hike in the afternoon. The kids need an activity break and it might give your host a break as well

- Tour the city –by foot or bike. Go to the city's downtown or Main Street. Even if you shop, you're still moving

FOOD FOR THOUGHT: You can't spot reduce. This would be nice. But you can't lose fat in one particular area of your body-just because you're working that part of your body. This means that you can do 1000 sit ups a day and it still won't get rid of the bulge around your mid-section. You can tone the muscle underneath, and your abs will get tight. However, the only way to burn the fat on top of the muscle, is to do aerobic activity and watch those calories.

Be specific with your exercise goals

Set goals that you can chart. If you're like most people, then you like to see numbers on yourself. We need to gauge our progress by giving ourselves specific numbers to achieve. For example, a goal could be… I want to be able to walk 15 minutes without stopping or breathing hard. Or I want to be able to participate in a line dance by the end of the year. Another goal may be that you want to jump one inch higher this year. Or you want to reduce your waist 5 inches by summer.

After your workout, take a ten second break and feel how invigorated your body feels. Feel your heart pumping, the blood pumping to the working muscles, and your body feeling a little tighter than before you started. It's a great feeling…and to quote a former baseball coach of mine, "nobody has ever drowned in their own sweat." That's right –it's OK to break a sweat –it's not going to kill you!

*"The greatest glory is not in never failing, but in rising up
every time we fall."*
-- Confucius

Exercise Hits and Myths

Over the years of training thousands of clients, I've heard plenty of myths
about why someone chooses to be active or why they don't. I'm going to
dispel some of the more common myths of exercising.

1. **No Pain, No Gain.** If you're in pain –you stop –NOW. Pain is
   your body's way of telling you that something is wrong. You
   don't have to work out that hard. Remember my motto, "train-
   don't strain."

2. **I Have to Be in Shape to Work Out.** You don't have to be in
   great shape to do any of my programs-just the desire. I just want
   you to move and stay active.

3. **I Cant Workout –I'm Too Old.** Being physically active will help
   you feel better –I don't care if you're 8 or 88. Your body was
   meant to move!

4. **More is Better.** I truly hope that you realize that moderate levels
   of exercise can produce some awesome health benefits. You
   don't have to become a bodybuilder or run a marathon to see
   results. Consistency is the key.

5. **People will make fun of me.** Do you think that all these exer-
   cisers started at their current level? No, believe me, we all start
   at different god-given skill levels, and even the most hard core
   fitness queen or king will tell you that they were awkward with
   the movements at first. Get out there and move. Trust me, if you
   go into a health club, no one's looking at you-they're too busy
   looking at themselves!!

6. **If an Exercise is Fun, then it's not Exercise.** Fitness should be
   something you enjoy and look forward to. I know you enjoy seeing the results-right ?

I'm a firm believer that if the exercise is fun, then it will lead to consistency.
Consistency beats out intensity any day of the week. You're in this for the

long-haul (your life) not a brief summer fling with fitness. Make fitness a priority – commit to it!

FOOD FOR THOUGHT: Did you know that your heart is your strongest muscle? It beats 100,000 times and pumps 2100 gallons of blood every day.

Be Sneaky...

Here are some simple ways on how you can fit more physical activity into your life...without even thinking about it.

1. Don't use the remote control on your TV or VCR - only your thumb gets a workout.

2. Store things in inconvenient, hard to reach places. This reaching works your back muscles.

3. Do your chores the old-fashioned way –without gadgets... dishwashers, food processors, and power motors. Our ancestors had the right idea.

4. Don't stack dishes on a tray when you clear the table –remove one at a time. Your guests and family will be impressed.

5. Use fewer wastebaskets at home. You'll have to walk more to fill them up –so why not?

6. Stand for an hour more every day. Standing burns more calories than sitting. I guarantee that you'll be more active –JUST by standing up. Your body will be in motion.

7. Place the laundry room on a different floor in your home. You'd be surprised how much of a workout carrying a load of laundry up and down the steps can be.

8. Use only one phone in the home. This will force you to get up and move! At our house, we like to have hand-held phones, so that we can stand up and move around while we talk.

9. Walk to the furthest bathroom –at a brisk pace-especially if you have to "go."

10. Carry the groceries to the car yourself. This really gives your upper body a workout. As you continue to do my exercise plan, you'll notice how much easier it is to carry the load.

STEP RIGHT UP!

I always recommend a pedometer to my clients. This tool allows you to measure your step-by-step process. You can gauge how much activity you really get on a daily basis. Are you moving or are you not? Let's find out. You may be surprised. Walking is one form of activity that is low–impact and is easy if you need to "ramp up " on your exercise program -- slowly.

STEP IN LINE

You can do daily activities to get your steps in during the course of a day.

Steps per minute

Mopping Floors	51
Gardening	73
Painting	78
Social Dancing	93

With your pedometer, walking ONE mile is approximately 2000 steps. According to the *America on the Move* program, the following chart gives you an idea of your current level of physical activity.

Very inactive	2500 steps or less per day
Inactive	2501-5000 steps per day
Moderately active	5001-7500 steps per day
Active	7500-10,000 steps per day
Very active	Greater than 10,000

From my own experience, if you're going to reach 10,000 steps during the course of a day, you'll have to add a formal walking/jogging plan to your schedule.

FEEL ENERGIZED!!

If you choose to purchase a pedometer, then I need your pedometer clicker to move-in order for you to reach your goals. If you don't Move – you don't Click – if you don't Click -You don't Lose!!

MOVE-CLICK-LOSE

FIT   HEALTHY   STRONG

VARIETY ...THE SEASONING OF YOUR MUSCLES

As in anything else –variety IS the spice of life. Please take advantage of our www.fit15.com website to receive a different circuit training routine everyday.

From this point on, consider the idea that your muscles are *smart*. When they do new things; whether it's dancing, martial arts, or strength training, they're a little shaky at first. They will learn quickly. By mastering these new moves, your muscles will become MORE efficient at doing them. So, they don't have to work as hard (or burn as many calories, or respond with positive gains) to keep up with the program.

For this reason, and the fact that you should always be challenging your body in order to keep improving your fitness level, you should deliberately alter your fitness routine "regularly." This can mean different things for different people. Some will alter their exercises on a daily or weekly basis. Whatever frequency you choose, change your resistance program at least once every 4-6 weeks. This change helps you to avoid hitting a plateau in the first place. On my plan, you can do this by altering the amount of weight you use for resistance.

SHAPE UP, SLIM DOWN, GET HEALTHY

Try this one out. I like to do this exercise while I'm doing nothing. This is a simple movement to tighten your abdominals (abs) without doing a sit up, especially if you're standing in line at a store, sitting at your desk or driving your car. Practice this move: Pull in your abs. Exhale and pull in your belly button as if you were trying to zip up a pair of jeans. Hold for 15 seconds and release-repeat as many times as you can.

Do what I do…Always keep your abs tight, chest out and back straight --- this **automatically** makes **you look leaner** and helps your posture.

"IN-DOOR" FUN/ENDORPHIN
Physical activity is a natural mood enhancer. The release of beta-endorphins is responsible for relaxing you and providing you with a sense of well-being–as in the "runners high."

IT MAKES YOU FEEL GOOD!

Visualize how your body will look when you reach your goal. Keep that image in your head –while you're working out or if you are tempted to skip your exercise sessions. It helps me to stay motivated on a daily basis. I truly believe that Fitness is the fountain of youth. Nothing staves off disease or growing old than a healthy commitment to an exercise routine.

FEEL ENERGIZED!

WHY BE FIT?

Here's a great list to motivate you every time you do any type of exercise. If I missed a few, sorry…but I think you get the point. Get up and Move-your body will thank you.

- Releases endorphins—and give you a feeling of well being

- Burns calories and fat-gives you muscles

- Lessens the chance of depression

- Regulates your appetite

- Encourages weight loss

- Raises self esteem, self confidence and self empowers you

- Boosts stamina

- Wards off Heart Disease

- Enhances your age

- Raises metabolism

- Keeps your heart and lungs healthy

- Prevents sprains, strains and day to day injuries

- Improves circulation

- Helps defend colds and flu's

- Decreases stress

- Increases energy, vitality and well-being

- Improves ratio of good (HDL) to bad (LDL) cholesterol

- Helps body make better use of insulin –reducing risk of Type 2 diabetes

- Improves lung function

- Strengthens bones –reducing risk of osteoporosis

- Reduces risk of osteoarthritis and osteoporosis

- Lessens lower back pain

- Improves muscular endurance

- Aids in digestion for optimal absorption of vital nutrients

- Helps to give you more quality sleep

- Slows aging process by improving blood circulation and delivery of nutrients

DAY 2
DAILY VICTORIES QUICK FIX: PERFECT PORTIONS

"Life's about choices, every time you choose a food that is nour-ishing– this moves you one step closer to your goal of being fit, healthy and strong"
- Anonymous

EXPANDING WAISTLINES

It's no secret that the American public is expanding their waistlines. In the past few years, the rise of obesity for adults has become a whopping one in two people. Bottom line…we're eating TOO much food.

Our lifestyles are partially to blame. Think about your own life right now. Do you eat on the run, eat at your desk or eat in front of the TV? Most of us take part in some, if not all of these behaviors. We eat out an average of four nights per week. And unless you are one to frequent nouvelle cuisine eateries, restaurant servings have made it impossible to eat normal portion sizes.

Super sizing has become the norm at restaurants; partly because of the need to keep up with the fast food mentality of more is better. Look around you, if it's not a value meal or a big gulp than it's a "grand meal."

Controlling portion sizes may be the single most effective thing you can do to promote lasting weight loss. Researchers have found that overweight individuals who spend the most effort controlling their portion sizes, are the most likely to lose weight. This is not only promoting healthy proportions of food, but this lean living will ensure that you keep the weight from returning.

NOTHING TASTES AS GOOD AS BEING LEAN FEELS

You have to want to be lean - more than you want to eat the wrong foods. It's <u>worth it</u> to make some sacrifices –controlling your portions and eating healthy!

Portion Power

I truly believe that after a few short weeks, you'll become a portion expert and you'll be able to "eyeball" your meals and determine the food quantity to ensure that you make weight a <u>non-issue</u> in your life.

An easy gauge to successful portion control will be determined by the way your clothes fit. In the first few weeks, you'll learn proper serving sizes by implementing your GET LEAN IN 15 menus, and paying close attention to the stated portion sizes. If you've been eating more than you should, then the pounds will start to creep up again. Remember the old adage, "your eyes are bigger than your stomach." If this does happen, then you know the foolproof method is to reintroduce the GET LEAN IN 15 plan into your life.

Once you get a sense of serving sizes, you'll be delighted with the results and satisfaction. You'll find that you can now control your weight and balance your nutritional budget without starving yourself or going on fad diets.

You'll find that it's easier to control your portions by using my patented LEAN PLATE at your home or office. This a great tool for you to use until you become an expert at judging correct serving sizes. The LEAN PLATE eliminates all the guesswork. You'll never have to weigh, count or measure calories again.

All these diets out there are confusing. Is it Low carb, No carb, Low fat, No fat… this should prove to you that **calories count no matter what** type of food it is. My menus include all foods –because variety is another key to long-term commitment. I have found that a failsafe way to ensure that you won't be tempted to overeat, is to eat the low calorie foods on your plate first; such as, salads, fruits, vegetables and soups. These foods will fill you up faster and not out. And save the meats and starches for last.

You may eat a few extra calories at one meal – knowing that you filled your plate with all your favorites – but guess what? It's O.K. Just be more aware at the next meal and make healthier choices and don't let that become a habit. If you're with a friend, then share your dessert or if you're alone, then eat half and save the rest for another day. If you're at someone's home for dinner, then insist that you "dish" out your own food. Don't be afraid to ask for a doggie bag at restaurants. Don't stuff yourself! Eat to the point of being satisfied, not stuffed and then ...**STOP!!** Portion control should be as natural as brushing your teeth.

VALUE YOURSELF, Not an Enormous Portion for the Buck

There are certainly times when more is better than less. However, when it comes to food and drinks, I can't think of too many occasions when it's better to consume more calories than you need. An extra 7 ounces of your meat is NOT A GOOD THING –three or four ounces is plenty. Remember, that's ounces –not pounds!

Restaurants and fast food places have all "upped" the ante with their portions and it should be no surprise that we've become a nation that is "oversized."

BIG PORTIONS = MEGA CALORIES

We as consumers want to have more bang for our buck. We equate portion size to value. Did you know that by eating an additional 10 fries per day or an ounce of cheese, which is approximately an extra 100 calories per day, can add up to a <u>10 pound</u> gain in one year. **CALORIES COUNT!!!**

Since more than 60 percent of the population of Americans are overweight; we clearly have a problem with portion distortion.
You can learn to moderate your portions by following these tips:

AT HOME:
- Use my LEAN PLATE -a portion control plate that eliminates guesswork

- Spread food across the table-if it's directly in front of you –you're more apt to nibble and pick up more food than you need

- Never taste while cooking – try chewing gum instead of testing the food

- Eat all meals sitting at the same place – preferably a table

- Never engage in other activities while eating (TV, reading) Studies have shown that you are oblivious to the extra calories being ingested

- Slow the pace of your eating. Instead of inhaling your food, enjoy the moment and put your fork down in between bites. Don't pick it up until you've swallowed the food in your mouth

- Increase the number of chews per mouthful –Gomer Pyle was right. His Grandma told him to chew more than 13 times for each bite

- Never eat out of the bag or carton, for it's extremely difficult to tell how much you're actually eating

- Use half as much oil as usual when you sauté vegetables for dinner tonight

- Drink half your pop now and half tomorrow- instead of downing the whole bottle in one sitting

AT THE STORE:

- Shop from your list and buy only those items on your list. This should eliminate temptations for the "extra" goodies. You have more control this way

- Shop after a full meal. I think this is self-explanatory. You will lose against the temptations of a grocery store. You're up against the food manufacturers and the aromas of the foods at the grocer are all triggering you to buy more food

AT THE RESTAURANT:

- Try ordering the lunch size portions. This size is probably as close as you're going to get to a proper serving size

- Share the meal with someone else

- Order water with lemon

- Ask for half or smaller portions- don't worry if it's not cost effective –it's worth it

- Eyeball your appropriate portion, set the rest aside, and ask for a doggie bag right away

- Use only half your normal creamer in your coffee-there's no calories in coffee –it's in the creamer

- Eat one slice of bread when making a sandwich instead of two slices. When I go to a restaurant, I do this quite a bit when I see that there's far too much bread with my sandwich

- Cut your mayo, oil based salad dressings and butter in half-these items are 100 % fat

These may sound like small things, but they really do matter in the big picture of forming healthy behaviors.

DON'T THINK YOU HAVE TO FINISH EVERYTHING ON YOUR PLATE!

My daughter Lauren is nine years old, and I have to constantly keep minding her to see how she eats. She grabs a bag of snacks and eats directly out of the bag. I think most kids do this, but they usually burn off these extra calories. Adults that continue this habit of eating out of the jar or the bag mindlessly, find it more difficult to burn these extra calories. Put your food in the bowl or plate. I promise you that you will have more control of your portions and still eat your favorites. Old Chinese saying "eat until you're eight-tenths full." Take heed of this –you don't have to finish everything on your plate –just because its there.

I DID IT: Success Stories with the LEAN Plate

JODI BEIGHT. 45 years old, mother of 1, lost 40 pounds. "The Plate made it simple and convenient to make sure I was getting all my fruits and vegetables for the day. I don't have to give up great tasting food with the Plate."

CINDY DETORE. 41 years old, mother of 2, lost 27 pounds, dropped 3 dress sizes. " I lost the weight without thinking of dieting – unlike other diets- my family can eat the same food."

PAM SLUGA. 41 years old, mother of 2, lost 28 pounds, dropped 4 sizes. "I can eat normal food and lose weight – without taking dangerous pills."

KIM BINNS. 39 years old, mother of 1, lost 37 pounds, dropped 4 dress sizes. "After a few months on the Plate, I learned to eat the correct portions for any meal – at home or in a restaurant, it came naturally because of the Plate. I've kept the weight off for 18 months."

SHARI PALUMBO. 42 years old, mother of 2, lost 37 pounds over the last 6 months, using the Plate for the past 2 months. "I love it. It has made eating much easier since I don't have to think about it."

DONNA ROSEN. 60 years old, Diabetic, lost a total of 150 pounds and over 40 total inches in 18 months with Jaime's products. Donna has had the Plate for 1 year. "I just love it. Before the Plate – I was eating way too much food for my needs – now I know how much food it takes to lose weight and keep it off."

ELAINE R. 48 years old, mother of 2, lost 24 pounds. "This is a great Plate for people to help them realize what a portion actually is."

PATTY M. 50 years old, mother of 3, minimal weight loss. " I liked it because it was real simple – a "no-brainer." I was enthralled with the different depth of the compartments. It helped me from overeating at my dinner meal."

CAROL D. 62 years old, mother of 3, post-menopausal, ex-smoker, lost 4 pounds in less than 2 weeks. "This was a "no-brainer"- just fill it up – it was easy."

HOLLY, lost total of 135 pounds – lost 50 pounds on the Plate " helped her break thru plateau."

Heather Kinder is a 25 year-old former client from Cleveland. She was miserable, desperate, and unhappy with herself for putting on the pounds. She told me that she would cry herself to sleep every night –wishing she were thin. She went on my plan and in 6 months, she dropped 65 pounds and 5 pant sizes. She is now loving life and very proud of her accomplishments…and she doesn't cry herself to sleep anymore.

Heather's not unique-it can happen to you too. HOW BAD DO YOU WANT IT?

The Fork and Spoon – Your Best Piece of Fitness Equipment

Diet Proof your Home

You might feel like grabbing "junk" once a day or several times a day. The urge might be at home, in the office or while you're driving. Identifying the environment and creating an obstacle between yourself and the "junk" will give you some time to get your thoughts back in order before you self-sabotage. These little diet alternatives will help you make better choices. Life's about choices…

In the KITCHEN:

High calorie snacks to keep OUT OF THE HOUSE	Fair Alternative
Ice cream	Frozen 8 oz cup of mixed yogurt
	Frozen yogurt tubes
	Sugar-Free Popsicles/Fudgecicles
Doughnuts	Whole wheat bagel with peanut butter
Cake	Sugar-Free Pudding w/ 1 % Milk
Pie	Sugar-Free Jell-O
Cookies	Graham Crackers
Other Pastries	
Butter Microwave popcorn	Smart pop Microwave popcorn
Chips	Baked Chips/Low fat Crackers
	Pretzels
Regular Pop	Diet pop
Kool-Aid or Juice Drinks	Sugar-Free Flavored Water
	100% juice
Alcohol	
Candy	

At the OFFICE

Watch out for:	Fair Alternative
Lounge	Packed lunch
Vending Machine	Fill Office Frig (fruit, yogurt, vegetables)
Candy on Desk	Bowl of Fruit on Desk
Cafeteria Dessert	Bottomless mug of Water

On the ROAD

In the Car, Stock

Stops to Avoid:	Fair Alternative
Fast Food	Ready to eat Fruit
Ice Cream Shop	Individual Bag of Pretzels
Big Gulps	Nutritional Bars
Gas Station Snacks	Can of Slim-Fast
	Diet Pop
	Bottled Water

Other Items

	Fair Alternative
Whole Milk	Skim or 1 % Milk
Full fat Yogurt	Low fat or Nonfat Yogurt
Toaster Pastries	Frozen Whole Wheat Waffles
Bacon	Canadian bacon
White Flour	Whole Wheat Flour
High-sugar Cereals	Oatmeal, whole-grain cereals or nuggets
Butter	Olive oil
Hard margarine	Soft tub margarine
High-fat salad dressings	Vinaigrette
Salt Shaker	Fresh herbs, DASH, lemon juice
Iceberg lettuce	Leaf lettuce, spinach, romaine
Convenience snacks	Fresh fruits and vegetables
Ice Cream	Frozen sorbet, frozen all-fruit
	Popsicles, fudgcicles

Portions and Proportions

Another key component to my plan is **PROPORTION**. The arrangement of your food is paramount for your success. This means that you need to balance the amount of protein, carbs, fiber, and fat that you are eating. This may sound complicated, but using the GET LEAN IN 15 system makes it easy.

The program's total calorie distribution is compliant with the recommendations from the American Diabetes Association, the American Dietetic Association, and the American Heart Association. Each menu has been planned to have approximately 55-60 percent of carbohydrate, 15-20 percent of protein and 25-30 percent of fat each day.

When I first started to devise this program, my simple rule was that if you looked at your plate, you should split it into fourths - quarter it. Three quarters would be fruits, vegetables, breads, cereals and grains and the other fourth would be lean protein.

All of the major health organizations agree on one thing: A diet that's high in fruits, vegetables, grains, beans and cereals and low in fat is essential to avoid chronic diseases like cancer, heart disease and stroke.

Eating most of these plant based foods cuts down on your saturated fats – which most guidelines tell you to limit. Moreover, if you want less fat on you –put less fat in you! Simple.

Balance, moderation and variety are the **KEY** to lifelong health and leanness. That's why when you follow my system, and fill your plate up with your favorite foods you ensure proper proportion as well as portion – guaranteed. The program is scientifically designed to give you an equal distribution of calories among meals to elevate your metabolism and help you burn more calories simply by doing what you truly love – **EATING!**

Who can remember each day whether or not they've had the proper amounts of servings? Five vegetables? Two milks? Six fibers? It's hard to keep track. Use the menus provided as your guide each day and before long –your food choices will become second nature to you.

Super sizing of America

According to a study from New York University, reports show that the standard size of foods such as burgers, fries, and candy bars has doubled since the foods were first introduced. It should come as no surprise that we as a nation are overweight - less movement + consuming more calories……..now that's an explosive combination.

Product and year it was introduced

		Max Size then	Max Size now
Canned Beer	1936	12 oz	24 oz
Bottled Beer	1976	7 oz	40 oz
Chocolate bar	1908	0.6 oz	8 oz
French fries	1954	2.6 oz	6.9 oz
Hamburger	1954	3.9 oz	12.6 oz
Soft drink	1954	12 oz	64 oz

The Journal of the American Medical Association did a study on the increase of portion sizes. The study found that between the years 1977 and 1996, each day we were eating:

93 more calories from salty snacks

49 more calories from soft drinks

97 more calories from hamburgers

68 calories from French fries

133 more calories from Mexican food

All these extra calories add up quick. So you can see how important it is to make sure your portions are correct. An extra 100 calories per day can turn into 10 pounds of FAT in one year.

Educating yourself on calories and portion sizes allows you to become aware of what's entering your body. This is more than half the battle. Also, show me the law that says you have to finish everything on your plate??

The following gives you a rule-of-thumb or hand (I mean this literally) for proper healthy serving sizes:

Pasta –1/2 cup   one cupped hand
Raw salad greens   two hands cupped together
Cheese   top half of your thumb joint
Fish (4 ounces)   little larger than the palm of your hand
Vegetables ½ cup   medium woman's hand
1 Teaspoon   woman's thumb
1 Tablespoon   3 thumb tips

80 % RULE

Eat until you're about 80 % full. Make a point of paying attention to the sensation of being full. Think of the word <u>SATISFACTION</u> – enjoy your food, without the obligation of cleaning your plate. Think <u>COMFORTABLE</u> –not FULL.

The **SMALL, SIMPLE** changes you make –have the **MOST DRAMATIC** and **LASTING** results

EAT LEAN -------------------------STAY LEAN

Real Life Portions

FOOD   SAME SIZE AS

<u>**Meat, Chicken, Turkey, Nuts**</u>

FOOD	SAME SIZE AS
3 oz cooked meat	Deck of Cards, your palm (a man's palm is closer to 6 ounces)
3 ounce grilled fish	checkbook
1-ounce sausage link	shotgun shell
2 tbsp Peanut Butter	ping-pong ball
1 ounce of nuts	one handful

Bread, Cereal, Rice and Pasta-starches

Pancake	compact disk
½ cooked Rice	a cupcake wrapper
½ cup spaghetti	fist
8 ounces lasagna	2 hockey pucks
½ cup mashed potatoes	½ apple
One small baked potato	computer mouse or Bar of soap
Slice of cake (3″ X 3″ slice)	Stack of Post-it notes
½ average size bagel	1 hockey puck

Vegetables

½ cup of steamed broccoli	light bulb
¾ cup of tomato juice	small Styrofoam cup
1-cup vegetable soup	baseball
1 cup salad greens	baseball

Fruit

½ cup of fresh fruit	7 cotton balls
¼ cup of raisins	large egg
medium size fruit	tennis ball

Dairy

1 ounce cheese	4 dice
1 tsp butter	tip of your thumb
1 cup of yogurt	tennis ball

Fats, Oils

1 tbsp dressing	1/2 golf ball
1 tsp butter margarine	size of a stamp or one die
Regular dressing 2 Tbsp	2 Tea bags
1 tsp vegetable oil	tip of your thumb

Snacks

1 ounce of chips or pretzels	two handfuls

DAY 3
DAILY VICTORIES QUICK FIX: Breaking the Label Code

"The journey from fat to fit – happens one pound at a time"
- Anonymous

Like most of us, you're probably baffled about how to actually decipher the nutrition labels on the back of food packages. However, in order for you to master the art of weight control, you need to be confident about using these labels to choose healthier foods. Without being a mathematician –I would like you to follow some basic "lean" guidelines as you begin to check these labels out.

Nutrition Facts

Serving Size 2 Crackers (14g)
Servings Per Container about 21

Amount Per Serving

Calories 60	Calories from Fat 15

	Daily Value*
Total Fat 1.5g	2%
Saturated Fat 0g	0%
Trans Fat	
Cholesterol 0mg	0%
Sodium 70mg	3%
Total Carbohydrates 10g	3%
Dietary Fiber Less that 1g	3%
Sugars 0g	
Protein 2g	

Vitamin A 0%	•	Vitamin C 0%
Calcium 0%	•	Iron 2%

*Percent Daily Values are based on a 2,000 calorie diet. Your daily values may be higher or lower depending on your calorie needs:

		Calories	2,000	2,500
Total Fat	Less than		66g	80g
Sat fat	Less than		20g	25g
Cholesterol	Less than		300mg	300mg
Sodium	Less than		2400mg	2400mg
Total Carbohydrate			300g	375g
Dietary Fiber			25g	30g

Start by looking at the serving size. This tells you a normal portion for this food. It is also the basis for all of the information on the label. In other words, all of the information on the food label pertains to the specified serving size, including calories, grams of fat, etc.... For this particular package, the serving size is 2 crackers. The next line then tells you how many of these "portions" are in this package–21 portions.

A common way that you may overeat is by consuming oversized portions and underestimating how many calories, fat, etc... are in the foods you eat. Don't feel bad. It's very easy to do. Please don't think that you can eat the whole box and JUST consume 60 calories. Let's do the math. First of all, I don't know too many people who are going to stop at eating just 2 crackers. Let's say you ate the whole box. That's 21 servings X 60 calories that's over a whopping 1200 calories! That makes a huge difference.

Don't eat the whole BOX!! To help avoid this, you might choose to buy single serving packages or remove a single serving from a larger package and put it in a bowl or on your plate.

If you would like to get more info on the entire label please go the following website: www.cfsan.fda.gov/~dms/foodlab.html

REAL LIFE for REAL RESULTS

Another important label fact that I look at is the **CALORIES FROM FAT** column. This will help you decipher the amount of fat a product has. Without being too complicated, I always follow this standard rule of thumb: For every **100 Calories** –you want only **3 TOTAL FAT GRAMS.**

Remember, there's 9 calories per one gram of fat. So, if we have 3 grams in a product that's 27 calories from fat. And if we know that the product has approximately 100 calories –than it's 27 % fat (100 divided by 27) also, keep in mind that unsaturated fats are healthier than saturated fats and trans fats. You want to keep your amount of **SATURATED FAT** at one-third your total fats or 10 percent.

Next look at the **FIBER** column. Foods that are usually high in fiber include fruits, vegetables, and whole grain products. And reading food labels can help you to choose foods that are high in fiber. A food high in fiber, like a can of vegetable soup, might have 4 or 5 grams of fiber per serving.

Understanding the **PERCENT DAILY VALUE** (DV) on a food label can help you choose foods that are high in good nutrients and low in bad nutrients. Remember, that 5 percent DV or less is low and 20 percent DV or more is high for a food component. For components like fat, saturated fat, trans fat, cholesterol, or sodium, look for foods with a low % DV. For these nutrients, you should try to eat less than the 100% DV.

And look for a high % DV for 'good things,' like dietary fiber, vitamin A, vitamin C, calcium, and iron.

An important fact to remember is that the % DV is based on a 2,000-calorie diet. Now, if you're following the GET LEAN IN 15 menu plans, they're based on 1200 calories. So, you can see how easy it is to eat more than you need. Also remember that the Percent Daily Values are listed for a single serving, so if you eat two servings, you should double % DV. Read the food label for specific serving size information. It's confusing-not everyone follows the same rules.... A serving of Cheerios is one cup, Kix makes a serving 1/3 cups and Great Grains granola is 2/3 cup.

The **INGREDIENTS** list is important because there are "hidden" ingredients that may not be on your list of healthy choices. The ingredients are ALWAYS listed by weight. The ingredients that weigh the most are listed first and down the list.

On the ingredients list, the first ingredient is about 80 percent to 85 percent of the total product by weight. Look for quality ingredients in the first three ingredients and that will be the bulk of the food. When you start reading the ingredient list you will learn a lot about your family's nutrition. If a food starts with sugar, salt or chemicals, bleached or enriched flours, you are basically getting nutritionally inferior products.

As stated earlier, with nearly two-thirds of Americans being overweight, one thing is for sure; we're eating too much! Ironically, America is also a society that is obsessed with being thin, and we spend tens of billions of dollars a year on dieting. Standard serving sizes are used by the USDA, but often for nutrition labeling purposes, the portion size is based on the unit or packaging. Always check to be sure the portion size you eat is based on your calorie needs.

Calculating your individual nutritional needs for weight maintenance and adjusting your diet accordingly is more effective than going solely by the standardized portions. In fact, depending on your diet needs, it may be OK to "eat twice the serving size" as long as you realize that you're eating twice the calories, protein, fat, etc.

Savor the Salt

The government has given us certain recommendations regarding sodium. The newly lowered guideline is now at 2300 milligrams, which is **about one teaspoon daily.** This is very easy to reach this level, so, it's important to avoid processed foods as much as possible. For instance, one can of soup easily contain almost half your daily dose of sodium.

At our home, we wash out all of our canned vegetables or beans. This eliminates some of the extra salt.

Selected High Sodium Foods...and Low Sodium Alternatives

INSTEAD OF HIGH SODIUM FOODS		TRY THESE ALTERNATIVES	
Food (serving size)	Amount of Sodium	Food (serving size)	Amount of Sodium
CONDIMENTS AND MISCELLANEOUS FOODS			
Baking powder, regular (1 teaspoon)	400-550 mg	Baking powder, low sodium (1 teaspoon)	5 mg
Baking soda, regular (1 teaspoon)	1370 mg		
Butter or margarine, regular (1 Tablespoon)	70-160 mg	Unsalted butter (1 Tablespoon)	0 mg
Garlic salt (1 teaspoon)	1480 mg	Garlic powder	1 mg
Pancake syrup (1 Tablespoon)	17-60 mg	Molasses (1 Tablespoon)	7-11 mg

INSTEAD OF HIGH SODIUM FOODS		TRY THESE ALTERNATIVES	
Food (serving size)	Amount of Sodium	Food (serving size)	Amount of Sodium
CANNED FOODS			
Regular pasta sauce (1/4 cup)	125-275 mg	Prego no salt added pasta sauce (1/4 cup)	25 mg
SNACK FOODS			
French fries (small order)	150-700 mg	Frozen, unsalted French fries (3 ounces)	10-20 mg
Nuts, dried & salted (1 ounce)	120-250 mg	Nuts, dried, unsalted (1 ounce)	3-10 mg
Nuts, honey roasted (1 ounce)	30-90 mg		
Popcorn, microwave (3 cups)	135-500 mg	Popcorn, air popped, unsalted (3 cups)	1 mg
Popcorn, oil popped (3 cups)	300 mg		
Potato chips (1 ounce)	170-300 mg	Unsalted potato chips, Tim's Cascade (1 ounce)	5 mg
Prepared baking mixes (1 cup)	1500 mg	Wheat flour (enriched white or whole wheat) (1 cup)	3-6 mg
Self-rising flour (1 cup)	1600 mg		

Pour some sugar on me

Sugar comes in many disguises by the manufacturers. So buyer beware ! They're constantly trying to trick us consumers. Foods with added sugars will list corn syrup, fruit juice concentrates, honey, molasses, etc. on their ingredient list. Ready for the "other" sugar names:

- Brown sugar
- Corn sweetener
- Dextrose
- Fructose
- Glucose
- High-fructose corn syrup
- Invert sugar
- Lactose
- Maltose
- Malt syrup
- Raw sugar
- Sucrose
- Sugar
- Syrup

Whole Lotta Grains

Try to look for whole grains, which are healthier and are preferred to white, refined grains. Whole grain foods should have one of the following whole grain ingredients listed as their first ingredient:

- Whole wheat

- Whole oats

- Brown rice

- Bulgur

- Graham flour

- Oatmeal

- Whole grain corn

- Whole rye

- Wild rice

This is a little deceiving............but, a food is **not made with whole grains** if it is labeled with the words such as multi-grain, 100% wheat, seven-grain, stone-ground, bran, or cracked wheat. You need to look for the word "whole."

LEAN ON ME

When I work with clients, I make them sign a contract with themselves –stating that they are responsible to make changes to see any results. I'm giving you direct strategies that you can employ. I need you to choose any 3 LEAN strategies that you can implement for the week:

- I will eat one meatless meal per week

- I will keep the freezer full of frozen vegetables

- I will eat the fruits and vegetables off my plate first

- I will double up on my dinner vegetables

- I will have a salad for lunch instead of fries

- I will limit my portions of high calorie foods such as ice cream or cake

- I will eat fruits instead of sweets

- I will skip seconds and get out the Tupperware.

- I will drink a glass of water BEFORE each meal

- I will not snack when watching TV

- I will not nibble while preparing food or when putting it away

- I will stop eating before I feel full

- I will divide up single serving portions ahead of time, in sealable bags

- I will read the packaging for the serving size and eat only one.

FOOD FOR THOUGHT: Eat to Lose! Your body gets hungry every 3 to 5 hours. Impulse eating, or bingeing, is usually a result of poor planning. If you eat at regular times and never let yourself get too hungry, you'll be less likely to overindulge. Try to eat at least four to five times a day. For example, breakfast, snack, lunch, snack, and dinner. Just three meals can work too, provided the meals are balanced, and your breakfast, lunch and dinner are roughly equal in calories. <u>Bottom line</u>: This is a very significant change. You can lose tremendous amounts of weight just by planning meals carefully and sticking to a regular mealtime schedule.

Day 4

DAILY VICTORIES QUICK FIX: Breakfast is for Weight Loss Champions!

*"The key to happiness is having dreams,
the key to success is making dreams come true"*
- Anonymous

We all know it, we've all heard it --but we all don't practice it on a daily basis. You **must eat breakfast if you're going to have a successful weight management plan**. The word itself should tell you everything. Break–Fast. Break the fast. If you're like the majority of most folks, you probably eat dinner anywhere between 5-8 pm on most nights. Let's do the math. For example, let's say you ate dinner last night at 6 pm. You woke up at 6 am a little hungry, (rightfully so –it's been a full 12 hours since you last ate) but decided not to eat breakfast because of time or maybe because you think you might lose weight faster if you don't eat. These calories that you "thought" you eliminated will usually more than catch up with you later in the day when you give in to binge eating temptations.

So you skip breakfast. It's now 12 o'clock lunchtime (18 hours since you've last eaten) –and you're starving –and you're on the prowl for anything you can get your hands on–like a ravenous tiger waiting to pounce. Now your head's pounding and you're a little delirious because you've run out of fuel and can't think straight.

The fuel that keeps our motors running is glucose. Your brain and your nervous system need glucose to work: that means walking, speaking, stretching, typing - any activity requires this fuel. If you don't supply it, your system resorts to finding stored carbs or it tries to turn fat into glucose. You need food quickly –so you might grab a choice that's not as healthy –but it's convenient.

Do you see what's happening here? You're setting yourself up for failure on two fronts. 1.) when you're starving, you're most likely going to choose an unhealthier choice, and 2.) your body shuts itself down, goes into its survival mode and automatically lowers your metabolism-COMPLETELY OPPOSITE OF WHAT YOU WANT.

EAT YOUR BREAKFAST!!!!!!!!!!!!!!

Your Mom always told you that breakfast was the most important meal of the day and guess what…she was right! Breakfast is your body's chance for an early morning refueling. Missing breakfast can lead to binging later in the day, missed nutrients, trouble concentrating and decreased energy. If you're not hungry in the morning start with something light such as a piece of fruit and whole-wheat toast. If you're on the run, grab a low-fat yogurt, cottage cheese, fruit, individual string cheese, and whole-grain waffle with peanut butter or ready-to-eat whole-grain breakfast cereal.

I always say…EAT EARLY-EAT OFTEN!

500 Club

In all my experience in helping people eat healthier, I've noticed that a "magic" calorie number is to keep the calories for one meal under 500. That's why the GET LEAN IN 15 menus are based on these figures. Here's a few quick 500 calorie Breakfasts that will help assist you in your planning.

Breakfast:		Calories
1 ¼ cup Multi-grain Cheerios or Bran Chex		250
1 cup Skim/1% milk		100
1 large Banana		<u>100</u>
	Calories:	450

Blend Together:		
1 cup Plain Yogurt		120
1 ¼ cup Whole Berries		60
1 large Banana		120
½ cup Skim/ 1 % milk		50
1 Granola Bar		<u>120</u>
	Calories:	470

1 Whole Wheat Bagel		200
2 T Low-fat Cream Cheese		45
1 ½ cup sliced Strawberries		120
1 cup Skim/1 % milk		<u>100</u>
	Calories:	465

2 Fried eggs		150
1 tsp oil/Butter		45
3 strips Bacon		100
1 slice Toast		80
1 tsp Butter/Margarine		<u>45</u>
	Calories:	420

Sausage Muffin w/egg		440
Coffee		0
2 Creams		<u>45</u>
	Calories:	485

The Brenkus BREAKFAST. I add fruit to my cereal every morning. It's an easy way to get one serving in quickly. I have grapes, raisins or blueberries. I also have a concoction that I created called "Yogurt Surprise" that combines plain non-fat yogurt with a little cereal, raisins, grapes and sliced almonds. It's all here folks; tasty, healthy, sweet, crunchy, chewy– you get it all. This is a great way to start the morning off.

Give it a try. It may take a few days for your body to adjust, but after awhile, you will begin to get hungry at breakfast time. In the long run, you will thank yourself for creating this good habit and you'll most likely eat fewer calories over the day because you'll be less likely to overeat or eat badly at other meals.

 Over the years, eggs have received a bad rap in the media. However, it has since been proven that they don't significantly raise your cholesterol or increase the chance of you getting heart disease. However, a new study published in the latest issue of the Journal of the American College of Nutrition, has shown that eggs have a 50 percent higher satiety index than other common breakfast foods. This means that you'll feel full longer when you eat eggs for breakfast. That's important if you're on a weight management plan. Eating eggs for breakfast instead of a bagel can reduce hunger and caloric intake both at lunchtime and over the next 24 hours.

EGGcellent…. Tip:
I have to share a trick that one of my personal training clients told me about. One of the quickest –non messiest, ways to cook eggs is to microwave Egg Beaters or egg whites in a bowl coated with non-stick cooking spray. They taste great and in 2 minutes you can have a high protein, low-fat meal. I have incorporated this method into my morning meals at least three times a week.

By the way, nothing prohibits you from eating any type of food for breakfast. If you want a piece of turkey or a bean salad –I don't know of any written rule that dictates your choices for a certain time of day.

DAY 5
DAILY VICTORIES QUICK FIX: SKIM TO SLIM

"The pleasure you get from life is equal to the attitude you put into it"

-Anonymous

The Scale Keeps Mooooving Down

Choose fat-free or 1 percent when eating dairy products. This really helps to cut out the saturated fat. This minor change to your daily dairy choice will pay dividends with your health and waist. You have four basic choices when you buy milk; whole, 2%, 1% or skim-now known as fat-free. I would like you to choose 1 % or skim because the fat content is much lower in these two choices (it is zero in fat-free milk). Our packaging experts have tried to pull another fast one on us by creating a deceiving milk carton. Let's take a look at the fat content for these four types of milk. I think you'll be amazed that 1% and 2% are a lot higher in fat than you expected.

Milk	Calories	Fat Grams	% Fat
Whole	150	8	48
2%	121	5	37
1%	105	2.6	22
Fat-Free	90	.6	0

Isn't that amazing? Your 2% actually comes in at 37% fat..........it pays to start investigating labels. And, if you choose fat-free over whole milk, those 60 less calories make a huge difference day in day out. In the course of the year, you would save 21,900 calories and 6 pounds of fat. Not to mention that the fat in milk is saturated or an unhealthy fat!

The dairy group provides us with protein, carbohydrate and important nutrients such as –calcium and vitamin D. Calcium, as well as vitamin D, is a must for good bone health. Of course, the obvious food, which is abundant in calcium, can be found down on the farm – from our friend -the cow.

Fitting in dairy is easy. You could add a 1-cup (8 ounce) serving of skim or 1 % milk to your breakfast meal and a ½ cup (4 ounce) serving to lunch and dinner meals. Another alternative is to try 100-calorie low-fat yogurt or homemade sugar-free pudding made with skim milk.

*If you are lactose intolerant, try Lactaid 100 Milk or Soymilk in the dairy aisle of your grocery store. Lactose intolerant people usually tolerate yogurt well also.

Dairy Do's

Calcium is a mineral necessary for strong teeth and bones and is readily available in dairy products. You don't have to go "cold turkey" when trying to rehab this food group, think in a stepwise approach: Replace whole fat with reduced fat, then, replace reduced fat with fat-free. Ultimately, you will be able to include all of the following with less resistance from your or your family's taste buds.

- Fat-Free Milk or 1 % Milk

- Nonfat Yogurt

- Sugar-free Homemade Pudding

- Nonfat Cottage Cheese

- Fat free or reduced fat Ricotta Cheese

- Fat Free or reduced fat American Cheese, 2 slices

- Skim Mozzarella Cheese, shredded

The Bare Bones on Calcium. Osteoporosis afflicts nearly 24 million Americans and results in 1.5 million bone fractures per year. One out of three women over 50 will suffer a vertebral fracture. This injury can cause the spine to collapse leading to a height as well as a postural problem. Severe back pain and breathing problems are common occurrences because of this skeletal change. I know if you've seen someone who has osteoporosis, you can't help but feel their pain. Adding resistance training staves off this awful problem. Women have 10-25% less bone in their skeleton than males during early development.

The loss of bone mass is sped up dramatically for the first 5 to 10 years after the onset of menopause because of a decrease in estrogen, a hormone that improves calcium absorption.

Adults average 400-600 mg of calcium intake daily and are encouraged to increase their intake to 1000 mg per day. Certainly, there are supplements that will provide you with enough calcium. But why buy pills – when you can get the calcium in "milk" for
Free!!

Sources of Calcium

Food	Calcium (mg)
Plain yogurt (8 ounces)	400
Salmon with bones (3 oz)	400
Skim Milk (1 cup)	300
Swiss cheese (1oz)	200
Calcium Fortified OJ (6oz)	200
Tofu (4oz)	150
Broccoli (1/2 cup)	47

RESPECT THY BODY

I love this quote. An anonymous author penned it…memorize it!

When you respect your body – you are in partnership with it. You become grounded in your physical body and all it has to offer.
Your body will honor you when you honor it!

Treat your body, as a structure worthy of respect and it will respond in kind. Abuse it or ignore it and it will break down in various ways until you learn the lesson of respect.

Day 6
DAILY VICTORIES QUICK FIX: LEAN PROTEIN

"Without challenge, there is no achievement. Accept the challenge so that you may feel the exhilaration of victory"
- Anonymous

The leaner the better. You get about the same amount of protein in a serving of chicken, beef, fish or pork, but depending on the cut of meat you can get a little fat or a lot of fat. So why not choose leaner cuts of meat to get your nourishing protein. Leaner cuts have less saturated fat or unhealthy fat as well as fewer calories. We normally make the protein section of our food choice the "main meal."

It doesn't matter if it's in a sandwich or on your dinner plate. Protein is the centerpiece. People have always come up to me and asked what I eat to stay so lean. I can tell you…. my protein choices have and will always remain….LEAN. Chicken, Fish, Turkey, Pork and lean cuts of Red Meat will give you a winning edge for a great body.

By providing nearly 20 percent of your calories from protein, your body will be able to preserve muscle while you lose fat. Muscle is what keeps your metabolism up; the more muscle you have, the more calories you'll burn off each day. In addition, I've provided a little protein at each meal that greatly extends the feeling of fullness between meals.

More Protein = Less Weight? Your friend lost 14 pounds in two weeks, her cholesterol dropped 50 points, she has unlimited energy – you tell her that's amazing! How'd she do it? She then proceeds to tell you that she has completely eliminated carbs from her diet. She eats bacon, steak, cheeses, and big juicy hamburgers – but throws away the bun.

Despite the hype of a very popular fad diet, that has been touting high protein –no carbs, the American Dietetic Association states that these "no carb" diets are nutritional disasters and in the long run can increase your risk of osteoporosis, kidney problems, fatigue and other health problems.

I'm not a big fan of high protein diet plans –intuitively, it doesn't make sense for proper health.

There's never been any documentation to prove that by cutting out complete food groups, your metabolism will go through the roof and you'll burn body fat while you sleep. When you eat fewer calories, you'll lose weight. That's it – simple science.

What's left when you're down to one food group: deprivation, boredom, fatigue and some *temporary* weight loss. You know that your weight is going to come back because you haven't learned anything about eating for the rest of your life.

Making healthy choices with balance, moderation and variety is the key to keeping energy at optimum levels and dropping inches. There is an easy calculation to check how much protein your body needs to function. On the average, the daily-recommended intake is about 0.8 grams of protein per kilogram of body weight. For example, a woman who weighs 50 kg (110 pounds) would require about 40 grams of protein per day. For an average sized man 70 kg (154 pounds), the daily protein intake should be 57 grams. As you can see, you don't need hordes of protein to be healthy. And any protein that's not expended through energy, gets stored as – guess what? -- **FAT!!**

Of course there are many types of protein for you to choose. I certainly believe it makes sense to eat the leanest variety. Chicken, fish and turkey are certainly some of the better choices. Skinless always – since most of the fat is stored in the skin.

> Turkey Breast with skin   - 38 % fat
> Turkey Breast without skin - 19 % fat

Beef has more fat than its protein counterparts – but you can still choose lean cuts. Loin cuts or round contain as few as 4 grams of fat per 3 ounce trimmed serving.

Great Cuts of Meat

	Calories	Total Fat	% Fat
Turkey Breast (skinless)	100	1	9%
Top Round Roast	100	2	18%
Chicken Breast	142	3	19%
Veal Leg	126	2.8	20%
Pork Tenderloin	139	4	26%
London Broil	167	6	32%

Not So Great

	Calories	Total Fat	% Fat
Chuck Roast	301	22.5	67 %
Corned Beef	316	25.8	74 %
Brisket	332	27.6	75 %
Ground (4 ounces)	** 351	30	77 %
Ribs – short	400	35.7	80 %
Hot Dog (Jumbo-2 oz)	190	18	85 %

** 4-ounce ground meat is equivalent to 3 ounces cooked

Buyer Beware. When choosing meats, make sure you don't get duped into the slick, manufacturing of the "97 % fat free." The packaging makes it sound like you're getting a very healthy, low fat version of your favorite type of meat. However, when you look closely – they are basing these numbers on the **WEIGHT** of the product – **NOT** the product content. Check the back of a 97 % fat- free Bologna package. You'll be surprised to find a very high fat content –when you do the math.

For example, you choose a Porterhouse steak that claims to be 91 percent fat-free on the package. Sounds great – but wait!   Three ounces of Porterhouse steak has approximately 254 calories and has 18 fat grams. Since we know that 1 gram of fat yields 9 calories, then we must calculate that there is 64 percent of the calories coming from fat (18 fat grams x 9= 162 divided by 254). So, where does the 91 percent come from? The Porterhouse is 9 % of fat weight - that means 91 % of the product is other than fat.

I know it's confusing and you think this is not fair – but the Government gives the manufacturers this right. Here are a few other packaging distortions. These products seem like they must be low fat, but they actually can contain many more fat grams and calories than are optimal:

Extra Lean – means no more than 5 grams of fat per 100 gram serving
Lean – means no more than 10 grams of fat per 100 gram serving
Less, Fewer, reduced – means at least 25 percent less of a given nutrient or calories than the comparison food
Light (fat)- means 50% or less of the fat than in the comparison food

Meat To Muscle

You need an adequate amount of protein in your diet each day to preserve muscle mass and keep your immune system strong. Another important function of the protein group is to delay hunger. Protein increases satiety or the feeling of fullness. By replacing high fat meats with lean meats, and using the bake, broil or grill methods, you stand to save _well over_ 200 calories per serving. This adds up to huge savings over the course of one year. 200 calories X 4 Fatty meats per week = 800 X 52 weeks –41,000 calories /3500 = 11 pounds of fat saved during that year.

Healthy choices

- Turkey Breast (no skin)
- Chicken Breast (no skin)
- Center Loin Pork/pork tenderloin
- Beef: Sirloin, flank steak, tenderloin, ground round
- Egg Whites or Egg Beaters

Don't forget about non-meat choices that are also good sources of protein:

- **soy foods (may also count as a starch)**
- **peanut butter**
- **beans, peas, lentils (also count as a starch)**

Seafood

Here's another trick to keeping lean on a weekly basis. Eat some type of FISH at least 2 meals per week. You have an unlimited amount of choices. Fish is usually very lean and the fat it does provide is a healthy fat or unsaturated fat. Notice the GET LEAN IN 15 Menus and you'll see this pattern. I always feel leaner and not stuffy after I have a meal with seafood.

Crab

Cod

Haddock

Flounder

Grouper

Halibut

Salmon (a little higher in fat…but a healthy one)

Swordfish

Tuna (fresh or canned in water)

Whitefish

Non-breaded Fish

Shrimp

Scallops

Legumes

Beans are a great source of protein and filled with plenty of fiber. What a great energy food. Beans fuel your system and keep you healthy. Don't forget to wash the beans out if you choose them from the can. Any bean is going to be a good choice.

Adzuki beans

Black beans

Chickpeas

Great Northern beans

Kidney beans

Lentils

Lima beans

Mung beans

Navy beans

Tofu

Tofu Treats

An alternative to eating meat is to enjoy the benefits of soy foods such as tofu. Twenty years ago, people were still associating tofu with hippie, communal type living and not very mainstream. You could only buy it at co-ops or health food stores. Now, every grocery chain in America has an abundant amount.

The great thing with tofu is that it takes the taste of whatever you're cooking it with – it virtually has no taste – but it's full of healthy fats and other important nutrients –which make it a very good choice if you need to lower your cholesterol level. You can slice it, dice it, or crumble it up in a variety of meal plans with the GET LEAN IN 15 menus. There are endless types of soy foods on the market today besides tofu. Make it a point to go out on a limb and try some of these products for a nice change!

Get L.E.A.N and stay lean. When I decided to write this book, I wanted the acronym L.E.A.N. to stand for Learn Everything About Nutrition. If you follow these principles I'm giving you about nutrition, you'll have the confidence to realize that these strategies are tried and true. You will learn to be Lean.

Day 7
DAILY VICTORIES QUICK FIX: WINNING AT LOSING

"Pride is a personal commitment.
It is an attitude which separates excellence from mediocrity"
- Anonymous

Why do some people succeed at weight loss and others –not so lucky? Your attitude towards change and commitment has a lot to do with it. There are many factors that weigh in this process. Remember those 6 steps to change in the beginning of this book? This will tell you your pledge of health and how your mind affects this process. I will show you ways that you can master the art of winning ….at losing.

WINNING WEIGHS

"I'm too fat"
"I'll never reach my goal"
"I can't do this"

STINKING THINKING. Sound familiar? self-criticism, self blame, negative expectations…. negative mind chatter happens to all of us. Not only do you have to create positive self talk language, but you have to STOP and redirect yourself when the negative chatter occurs.

Being successful starts in your mind. Try to imagine yourself smacking into a huge red STOP sign when you find yourself thinking negatively about yourself. You will be forced to take another direction……choose a positive one. Being positive is a habit. You need to spend time and energy being positive. See, weight control isn't just about calories and exercise. You MUST determine to be positive regardless of what happens.

VISUALIZATION. Imagining is one of the most powerful ways to make your weight loss a success. Top professional and Olympic athletes use this. They use this to actually see themselves performing their event or sinking the winning basket. Just ask Michael Jordan how many times he saw the ball go through the hoop before he shot it.....I think you already know the answer.

Every minute of every day you have a choice to visualize the picture of success that you want. I want you to take a few minutes sometime today and use an <u>image of success</u>…of you having fun…staying relaxed.

Now, visualize yourself at your goal weight. Experience victory! See yourself walking with a friend or your spouse in one of your favorite places, maybe with a new outfit on. See how your body has changed… all the positive physical changes that have occurred since you started the program. You must think of this end result in terms of a very <u>present</u> possibility. You must see the possibility of your goal so clearly that it actually becomes real to you… so real that you feel the same feelings you'd expect to feel at your goal weight.

- **<u>Believe It</u>**-you can do what you see yourself doing in the minds eye

- **<u>Want It</u>** –desire is the fuel that sustains you

- **<u>Feel It</u>**-the greater the detail—the more effective the image will be

- **<u>Expect It</u>**-knowing that your efforts will pay off

- **<u>Be Specific</u>**- know what you want –know your goal weight

- **<u>Be Positive</u>**- use images and words to promote your success

Positive mind chatter…
- **"I'm full of energy today"**
- **"I feel I'm taking good care of myself"**
- **"I am proud of myself for eating well"**
- **"I am following my doctor's advice"**

Remember…. You are what you think!!!!!

FOOD FOR THOUGHT: **<u>If They Could See Me Now.</u>** I want you to write down on a piece of paper the healthy changes you're planning to make. You must have your goals and resolutions clear in your mind. Mark down the date one year from today.

Now, shut your eyes, and imagine that it's exactly one year from today. I want you to focus on all your health gains. What do you look like? What have you done that you're proud of? How do you feel? How would you describe the new you?

Keep replaying this positive picture in your mind. Make a habit of seeing you succeed! Think of how your life would change if you only had positive thoughts about yourself. You have the power to create your own reality. I want you to take a couple of minutes and write down some positive statements you can say about yourself. "I'm pretty, I'm a great mother, or great father, and I have high virtues." You get the picture. Visualization is a powerful way to achieve that positive attitude.

Don't just think you can wish it to happen. A wish is just what it is …a dream. If it's going to happen –you need to provide some action with that wish.

<u>IF –THEN SCENARIO</u>

Have you ever tried to lose weight before or set any other goal for yourself, and got caught up with the "if-then" situation. You'll find yourself thinking…

- **<u>If</u>** I lose 25 pounds, **<u>then,</u>** I'll treat myself to that cruise I promised myself

- **<u>If</u>** I get into a size 8, **<u>then,</u>** I'll go dancing

- **<u>If</u>** I get down to my High School weight, **<u>then,</u>** I'll go to the reunion

The problem with this thinking is that you're constantly "stuck" in a holding pattern. You're not feeling good about yourself right now, and waiting for magic to strike. CHANGE doesn't happen while you're waiting. Feel good about the process and reward yourself often. Don't wait to give yourself positive feedback.

I used to teach a weight management lecture focusing on positive mental attitude toward our bodies—NO MATTER WHAT SIZE we are………we're all just "average" bodies.

I would have the class say this credo out loud. We can all learn from this little lesson:

- I accept my body as uniquely beautiful because it's a part of me

- I do my best to be caring and nurturing of my body -as I would anything I love

- I don't expect my body to be perfect---I will allow myself to be average

- I will separate media and social messages that imply there's something wrong with my body

- I will recognize the health issues of my body and pursue solutions

*********I AM NOT JUST A BODY*********

Sweet Emotion

We all have the physiological need to eat. Why do some of us overeat …even when we're full? It's called emotional eating. Most people learn early in life that foods often serve other purposes besides nutrition. Let's face it, food is comforting. People eat for many reasons…. to reward themselves, celebrate occasions, and entertain others. People also eat to calm their nerves, eat out of boredom, eat because of rejection or sorrow. You name it….the list can go on and on.

Write On

I've found while working with clients that a sound way to untangle emotional triggers with food is writing down your thoughts. Make a point to include how you feel when you're eating. You will discover patterns that reveal the emotional cues that cause you to turn to food and possibly overeat. When you think that you're eating out of emotion, remember these two questions:

Sometimes I feel _____ when I'm eating

I usually feel_____when I reach for snacks

Eating for other Reasons

1. Emotional Rescue. Once you track down a problem – try to find an alternative to eating that will soothe your emotions. If you eat out of anger – call a friend to vent your frustrations. If you're lonely, reach out to other people- join a health club. Figure out whether your concerns about weight could be substituting for other unmet needs.

2. Please Release Me. When you're stressed out, you may eat or make unhealthy choices. Simplify your life. Share and delegate responsibilities. Save your energy for the most important people and activities - set priorities.

3. To Do or not to Do. Time management is important to alleviate stress. Get organized and make a daily "to do" list. Keep it realistic and don't try to cram in too many activities. It's OK to say NO to people.

4. Eat the Foods you Love – Lose the Weight you Hate. If you deprive yourself of your favorite foods–you're setting yourself up for failure. Deprivation will make you unhappy –which in turn could make you overindulge.

Foundation

Your foundation helps you feel connected to others – it goes beyond friendship. It's the "glue" that motivates people to act out of a sense of higher purpose or a dedication to something bigger. Having an inner-peace gives you a better sense of well being, higher life satisfaction, lower anxiety, and better coping ability- you feel grounded.

1. **Sound of silence**. Spend some time being – silent. Pay attention to where your mind goes when you're silent. This will help you get to know the "real" you.

2. **Drop in – tune out**. Avoid always turning on the TV or Radio. Get rid of some of these outside distractions that can make you less peaceful or unproductive.

3. **Don't despair – don't compare**. You're an individual – you don't have to be like anyone else. You don't have to measure up to anyone. Understand this emotion and it will help set you free with yourself. Console yourself with the fact that almost all women and even men, thin or not, are unhappy with some parts of their bodies.

4. **Here comes the Judge.** Always be kind to yourself and don't judge yourself. No one is perfect. You're not supposed to be. You can handle the good as well as the bad – because you're strong.

POSITIVE DIRECTION

Watch your BODY Language

I have learned working with clients over the years that most people would rather look for the negative aspects about themselves and focus on those. Try and discover what factors play a role in your struggle with your body. Create a Lean lifestyle that increases your chances for ending this war with your body- NOW. Years in years of this mind battering tend to wear you down and dim your hopes. Let's try a few small things that will help you move in a more positive direction.

1. Look in the mirror as a whole person –rather than a collection of parts. ***note the parts that you feel are attractive. C'mon I know there a few things that you like!

2. Get in touch with your body sensations during a physical activity you enjoy. **Note the way your body is moving and feeling. This helps you gain confidence that your program is working- YOU WILL FEEL BETTER.

3. Take care of all aspects of your body---teeth, nails, hair, eyes, skin, etc... ***note the aspects of your body that you can change immediately to make you feel good. We love instant changes –this is no different –think how good you feel after a nice haircut or a trip to the beauty shop.

4. Seek out all the people who are positive and non-judgmental about their appearance and the appearance of others. ***Note a few people you can turn to for positive stimulation. You'll be surprised how this frees you up and lessens the pressure of trying to compete with the next body that walks by.

5. Try on clothes in your new size. Keep one "fat outfit" for comparison. Wear clothes that allow you to move freely: flat, comfortable shoes, flowing skirts, and stretchy fabric. Don't worry about the size – but how it fits and how it makes you feel. Do me a favor-this is money well spent-buy a pair of jeans that are a few sizes two small. Try them on every few weeks. You'll be amazed how your body changes and is reshaped from my plan.

6. Pay attention to how you fit into spaces. **Note how you fit into chairs, behind the steering wheel, through doorways, etc...this will help you gauge your success –when you can fit into spaces more easily and less cramped.

7. Visualize yourself thin. **Take a moment right now and shut your eyes and dream what you want to realistically look like. Go ahead ...it's free, fun and fantastic to let go and envision the future. Keep in mind, when you think of beauties like Marilyn Monroe, Sophia Loren and Raquel Welch – these women had shoulders, and breasts and hips and are considered the sexiest women ever seen.

8. Make appearance less important by developing other benchmarks for self-evaluation. Focus on succeeding at work, playing sports, friendships. Practice using your body to do something-plant a garden, build a shed, have a baby, instead of treating it as an object to be stared at.

9. Imagine yourself successful – and you'll be successful. Imagine yourself a failure – and you'll probably fail.

CELEBRATE YOURSELF!!

SHOWING IT OFF!

FOOD FOR THOUGHT: I feel healthy, I feel happy, I feel terrific!

---

1. You can control your mental attitude by the use of self-motivators. Use self-motivators such as "I feel healthy, I feel happy, I feel terrific" to motivate yourself to positive action in the desired direction. It sounds quirky and flaky –but I don't think you can deny –it makes you feel better than knocking yourself down on a daily basis.

2. If you set a goal, you are more apt to recognize things that will help you achieve it than if you don't set a goal. Keep trying until you hit it. And the higher you set a goal, the greater will be your achievement with positive mental attitude. AIM HIGH!

3. To succeed in anything, it is necessary to know the rules and understand how to apply them. It is necessary to engage in constructive thinking, study, learning and planning time with regularity. Study your work well-apply techniques and do them well enough that they become natural. Eating right, thinking lean and exercising should become second nature to you…it is NOW your lifestyle –you own it!

No matter what you do —you owe it to yourself to find satisfaction in your life. Satisfaction is a mental attitude. Your own mental attitude is the one thing YOU possess over which you alone have complete control.

WHAT THE MIND CAN CONCEIVE AND BELIEVE, THE MIND OF MAN CAN ACHIEVE

When it comes to your health . . . it's all about you.

Negative Mind Chatter

Do you recognize any of the following negative thought habits?? This will help you establish what negativity looks like when it raises its ugly head. Move it out –and keep it out ....NOW!

1. **Criticism-** thinking over and over how badly you did. How about saying –I did the best I could for now. Next time I'll do even better.
2. **Blame-**telling yourself you're responsible for situations actually beyond your control. Try not to dwell on these situations ...they soon shall pass and you can gain control the next meal or next day to exercise.
3. **Negative Expectations-** always dwelling on the worst that could happen. I know this is tough not to replay old messages –but this is a doable program –that you can and WILL stick with.
4. **Should** – always telling yourself what you ought to be doing – even if it's unrealistic. This is the time to cease the action and start becoming proactive. I should've done this –I should've done that –if it's going to help you get to your goal-pull yourself together and do it ...Now.
5. **Can't** – believing you can't do something-when it's actually within your capabilities. What part of eating right or exercising regularly can't you do?? Here's a perfect example of erasing that word. I truly had people come up to me and say you CAN'T write a book –you don't know how to write. Well, wonder if I listened to them –I wouldn't be helping you right now. P.S. I autographed a copy of the book for them...and it felt GREAT!!

When you find that you're feeling badly about yourself – ask yourself ....What beliefs am I acting on ? What has my self-talk been that has produced such feelings? What negative thought pattern have I slipped into?

SAY the RIGHT things to yourself.
1. Make a firm decision to change.
2. Become aware of the irrational or negative thought ---identify it.
3. Take time to ponder that negative thought.

Being POSITIVE is a HABIT. You need to spend time and energy practicing being positive. We MUST determine to be positive regardless of what happens. Remember that habits are not easily broken. Remember to act ONLY on Principle — according to what you know to be right –even if you don't feel like it. Your feelings will soon catch up. **Fake it till you make it!**

I always say...........

YOU NEVER FAIL --UNLESS YOU STOP TRYING!

One of the most important keys to life-long weight management is self-esteem. Some people have a low self-esteem because they're overweight. Others become overweight because of low self-esteem. This scenario forms a VICIOUS CYCLE

"I'm overweight, therefore, I might as well eat a whole pizza to make myself feel better, therefore, I gain even more weight, and therefore, I feel even worse about myself."

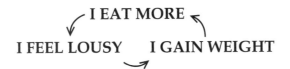

The first step is to learn to accept yourself as you are. Realize you're still a worthwhile, good person even if you don't lose an ounce.

YOU DON'T NEED TO BE SKINNY TO LOOK GREAT

Dump the Doubt

I can't do this-I can't stick with this –there's no way I can live like this the rest of my life. Oh, these words can tear us apart. Do you want to hold up your progression towards a healthy lifestyle? The best saboteur of your goals is to have doubt. Yet doubt is nothing but a thought, and has no power other than the power you give to it. You have the authority and control to let go of this albatross. Any doubt, with a little mental effort, can be vanished the very second you want it to.

All doubt is yours by choice. Yet when you simply let it go, the doubt falls away from you and rapidly dribbles into nothing. There's not one single doubt that is permanently affixed to you. Fill your mental computer chip with positive, empowering confidence that you can…. and will make the necessary changes for life lasting health. There's a solution for everything…if you want one!

TAKE CHARGE NOW

Your outlook and attitude towards your self will determine how successful my plan will work for you.

I hope you can answer **YES** to most of these statements:

- I do my exercises –even when I don't feel like getting active

- I know I can keep this lifestyle up if I WANT TO

- I am the only one who can decide be active or be a couch potato

- I make commitments to eat healthy on a daily basis and then I fulfill them

- I schedule exercise on a regular basis

- I am proud of the way I am approaching my healthy lifestyle

- I don't let other issues affect my healthy lifestyle

- I don't make excuses for not being active

- I like when other people admire my new lifestyle

Day 8
DAILY VICTORIES QUICK FIX: Go Green

"Cherish your visions and your dreams as they are the children of your soul; the blueprint of your ultimate achievements"
-Anonymous

As you will see with your **GET LEAN IN 15** menus, you will be eating something green twice a day. This was not a misprint. The reason is simple; vegetables are one of the secrets to eating your way to **YOUR** best figure. Power packed with nutrients and very few calories, the more vegetables you eat, the healthier and thinner you become – case closed.

Salads and green vegetables are chock full of fiber and increase your feeling of fullness. At my house, I start every dinner with a salad and vinaigrette. Eating a salad first lessens the chance of gorging the entire meal, because I don't have to eat seconds or feel the need for extra goodies. You want to get lean and stay lean …take heed of this Daily Victory …and Go Green everyday.

Life's about choices !

Again, you can get your vegetables through a variety of ways; fresh, frozen or canned. At our home, we rinse all the canned vegetables, since they are usually very high in sodium. I'd recommend that you do the same. When it comes to produce, variety is the key to getting all your vitamins and nutrients from this food group – and it's more fun than just eating the same vegetables week in /week out - mix up the colors!

These are some ways to eat healthier quickly:

- Ready to eat bags of salad. My family utilizes these bags every night. You may call it lazy. I call it smart

- Use a microwave to quickly "zap" vegetables. This helps you with the preparation time…I love the way broccoli looks after you microwave it. It's dark green and exudes health …give me more please! Microwaving or steaming vegetables with just a small amount of water preserves more of the nutrients then boiling them to mush

- We usually add frozen vegetables to any pasta dish. It's an easy way to get in another serving of the good stuff

- Buy canned vegetables labeled "no salt added" and throw them on top of your salad or on your plate with low-fat vinaigrette

- Many vegetables taste great with a dip or dressing. Try a low-fat salad dressing with raw broccoli, red and green peppers, celery sticks or cauliflower

- Keep a bowl of cut-up vegetables in a see-through container in the refrigerator. Carrot and celery sticks are traditional, but consider broccoli floret's, cucumber slices, or red or green pepper strips. We also buy the carrots that are already shredded - it makes it so convenient to throw them on our salad. We also include sun-dried tomatoes or the little cherry tomatoes on the salad. It's an easy way to get more healthy nutrients and fiber to your diet

I know sometimes it's difficult to stick to new eating habits. But, you'll have to realize that ONLY YOU have the power to decide what to eat everyday. No one is forcing you to eat a certain type of food. If you're devoted to living a life of "leanness," than you will stick with eating a few more vegetables every day.

When in doubt, always opt for brighter color food. It's been my experience that most high-calorie, high-fat menu items are brown, beige, white or pale yellow. I always tell me daughter, Lauren, to think of adding color to her plate. I want to see a rainbow on her plate…. and yours.

Green Lean Machine

Look for the darker colored vegetables; they are more nutritious. Beta-carotene, most strongly noted for its suppression of certain types of cancers and it's protective properties against heart disease, is most commonly found in plant foods that are orange, red, dark yellow and some that are dark green. Think about the color of your lettuce choices. Romaine, spinach, spring mix or kale has more nutrition and is higher in fiber than iceberg lettuce, because of its rich green color.

Produce is a great way to increase the fiber in your diet and pack your body full of antioxidants to help ward off cancer and heart disease as well as many other medical issues. Why not choose these deeper colored choices …they're worth the extra money. Your health is worth it.

Produce to Reduce

Vegetables are in a similar family to the fruits. Because of the high water and fiber content of this food group, the "dieter" feels full longer with delayed gastric emptying and a sense of heightened hydration. The additional antioxidants support better vision and healthier skin. Also, if you find yourself feeling a little less full than you'd like on my menus, add a side salad to the meal. You can use regular dressing of your choice if you dip the fork on the side. Otherwise, use a fat-free dressing, flavored vinegar, or squeeze some lemon. ALL vegetables are really low in calories. They would make my "free" list of foods-foods that you could eat anytime in any amount. I don't know too many people who can sit down and eat two heaping plates full of broccoli.

To create your salads from my menus, choose from this
COMPLIMENTARY VEGETABLE LIST:

lettuce	radish	cucumber	sauerkraut
broccoli	cauliflower	carrots	spinach
cabbage	celery	tomato	peppers
green beans	asparagus	pickles	waxed beans
bean sprouts	onion	mushrooms	alfalfa sprouts
beets	turnips	zucchini	pea pods
eggplant	greens	okra	water chestnuts

Think Color

GREEN - Full of folacin for healthy blood...and fiber for a healthy bowel

Broccoli

Peppers

Dark leaf lettuce

Zucchini

Spinach

Asparagus

Beans

Peas

Kiwi

Grapes

YELLOW – Doses of Vitamin C, Vitamin A and Potassium

Squash

Lemons

Pears

Bananas

Mangoes

ORANGE – Full of Vitamin A for healthy vision and Beta Carotene for anti-aging

Carrots

Cantaloupe

Sweet Potato

Oranges

Tangerines

RED – Doses of Vitamin C for a strong immune system, healthy skin and gums

  Tomatoes

  Strawberries

  Peppers

  Red Potatoes

  Grapes

 FOOD FOR HEALTH: If you don't have time to wash or chop — POUR yourself a little health. Six ounces of vegetable juice equals one serving of vegetables.

The Brenkus Household

For years, clients would always want to know what's in my refrigerator and pantry. I believe that I have followed guidelines that are conducive to a lifestyle of leanness. Come over and take a look…………..

MEATS

  Turkey Breast slices

  Hummus

  Chicken slices

  Salmon

  Olives

GRAINS/BREADS/CEREALS

100 % Whole Grain bread

Whole wheat Pita

Instant Brown Rice

Oatmeal

Baked Tortilla chips

Couscous

Whole Grain crackers

Angel Hair Pasta

Kashi cereal

CUPBOARD

Air-popped popcorn

Lite Chocolate Syrup

Herb Tea

Fig Bars

Almonds

100% fruit preserve

Raisins

Tomato Sauce

Canned or packets of water-packed Tuna

Salmon packets

Applesauce

Peanut Butter –natural if possible

Olive Oil

Low-sodium Vegetable Soup

Reduced Fat Chicken Soup

Chocolate (my wife's and daughter's)

DAIRY

Skim Milk

Low-fat Cottage Cheese

Non-fat Plain yogurt

Part Skim ricotta cheese

Egg Beaters/Egg Whites

Reduced-calorie Margarine – Smart Beat

BEVERAGES

Bottled water

Orange juice

Diet soda

VEGETABLES

Ready to eat salad

Broccoli

Carrots

Cherry tomatoes

Peppers

FRUIT

Granny Smith apples

Oranges

Nectarines (or any seasonal fruit)

Day 9
DAILY VICTORIES QUICK FIX: Drink to Victory

"Don't wait for your ship to come in – swim out to it! There is an island of opportunity in the middle of every difficulty"
- Anonymous

I would rather you EAT your calories then DRINK them. Here's why— you'll feel more satisfied. With food, at least you're getting the satisfaction of chewing and tasting your calories and therefore, you have a better chance to know when you're full.

I have found with my clients that because you normally don't associate beverages with high calories and fat –that it's OK for you to guzzle as much as you want …without harm or consequences.

Wow! That's the furthest from the truth. Calories count no matter what source. Many beverages sneak on the pounds very quickly without you being totally aware of their damage. I'm going to be blunt here. IF YOU WANT TO SUCCEED TO BECOME LEAN …LEARN TO LOVE WATER.

I know you always hear you need to drink eight 8-ounce glasses of water a day for better health. I don't disagree –but I don't want you to be locked in to a specific number. I think it's extremely important to realize that there are foods that have high water content and there are other beverages that are water based like teas that hydrate you just as well.

This may sound crass. But here's my simple plan to tell you if you're drinking enough liquids. Check the color of your urine. That's right. If it's clear or slightly pale yellow, then, you're drinking enough water – keep up the good work. If it's dark yellow ….then sprint to the nearest water fountain. This is a real good indicator, and it doesn't have to be determined by a set number of glasses per day. Also, I want to remind you that if you're taking a multi-vitamin supplement, this will make your urine bright yellow shortly after taking it, so you may not be able to use this test at all times.

Drink water throughout the day. You don't hear this nearly enough: water is an all-purpose wonder-substance. It's great for your skin, your digestive system, and circulatory system, and aids in weight loss and cellulite reduction. If you feel fatigued during the day, it's often because you aren't hydrated properly. Drink water throughout the day, fill up a large bottle early in the morning and make sure by the end of the night that you've finished it. If you have it nearby, it's easy to remember.

I never met a water faucet that I didn't like. I make it a point to visit most water faucets that I pass. Wet your whistle often and you'll get in the habit of enjoying the results that water can do for you. (Try not to touch the faucet with your mouth –I'll reserve comments for a future book)

If you really don't like the "taste" of water, squeeze a little lemon juice in there. This should help. There are flavored waters now popping up in the marketplace. However, make sure that it's just water and a little flavoring and NOT flavored with some type of sugar….that means that there's plenty of calories –you don't need.

Don't keep an endless supply of soda in the fridge. Buy only enough to have one a day, and ration it out. Regular soda provides a lot of calories, all in the form of sugar. If you choose soda at all, go for the diet version! I don't have a problem of you drinking Diet Sodas from a calorie count –they certainly fit into the equation. However, these sodas may not re-hydrate you as properly as water.

Try replacing soda with water or unsweetened iced tea for just a week — then have a can. You may be surprised to find you've lost the taste for it!

Stop drinking soda out of a can. Instead, fill a glass with ice, and then add the soda. You'll drink less soda, and it will be easier to eventually wean yourself off it.

Calculate the calories. If you drink one soda a day for a year, that's 58,400 calories, or almost 17 pounds from the can… ouch!

 FOOD FOR THOUGHT: H2O to Go! If you drink water for lunch and dinner –instead of pop or alcohol –you will lose 7-15 pounds in one year.

Beer Bells (not barbells)

Ah yes, the 12-ounce curls. Not only does alcohol contain 7 calories per gram, but it also lowers self-control when it comes to food. Studies have shown that when you drink alcohol before or during a meal, it lowers inhibitions and control when it comes to eating, causing people to eat more than those who waited to drink after finishing a meal.

All alcohol has plenty of calories, but beer remains one of the best choices regarding caloric intake. The most common beers have between 100 –120 calories per beer. Light beers can be as low as 90 calories per 12 ounce. A 3.5-ounce of wine and a shot of liquor have approximately 100 calories also. Fruity tropical drinks could have more than 300 calories per drink. Alcohol has no fat in it. However, the empty calories (EC's) add up quick and like always, these "EC's" put on the pounds when not burned off.

The list below breaks down the number of calories in typical alcoholic drinks. Compare some of your favorites to make a good choice next time you decide to indulge in a serving of alcohol.

Drink	Serving Size	Calories
Red wine	5 oz.	100
White wine	5 oz.	100
Champagne	5 oz.	130
Light beer	12 oz.	105
Regular beer	12 oz.	140
Dark beer	12 oz.	170
Cosmopolitan	3 oz.	165
Martini	3 oz.	205
Long Island iced tea	8 oz.	400
Gin & Tonic	8 oz.	175
Rum & Soda	8 oz.	180
Margarita	8 oz.	200
Whiskey Sour	4 oz.	200

A helpful hint for saving some calories for the week…Limit alcohol to weekends.

SQUEEZE ME. I know that most people would truly believe that drinking juice would be a much healthier choice than a soda pop. I would agree that juice has more healthy nutrients. But what you probably didn't realize…Juice has as many calories, ounce for ounce, as soda. So, as in anything else I've told you -moderation is still the key. Set a limit of one 8-oz glass of fruit juice a day and you should be OK. Dilute your juice with water. Juice is sneaky – a 16-ounce cranberry-grape blend contains 340 calories.

Day 10
DAILY VICTORIES QUICK FIX: Do The Dip

"The important thing is this; to be able at any moment to give up what we are- for what we can become"
– Charles Dubois

You may think this is an odd action plan. However, I've found that people don't realize how calories can secretly creep up very innocently. The fat of dressings and oils adds up quickly and can sabotage your weight control plan quicker than you can say, "I'll have Ranch -please."

Have you ever heard anyone or maybe you've said this yourself..."I don't know why I can't seem to lose weight- that's all I do is eat salads." It's not the salad that packs on the pounds – IT'S THE DRESSING!! A regular size salad with lettuce, carrots and a few tomatoes only has 50 calories. The dressing, which is oil based, has about 120 calories per tablespoon. Now, who stops at one tablespoon? Let's do the math. It's safe to say, that it's very simple to pour on the dressing and get as many as four or five tablespoons of dressing on your salad.

5 X 120 calories=600 CALORIES
           with almost 100 percent coming from fat!

That once low calorie choice has now become a very HIGH FAT choice, and will most assuredly sabotage your lean eating plan. Given that the average serving of dressing on a salad at a restaurant is ¼ cup, you stand to spare yourself over 40 pounds of body fat over the next 10 years. And that's if you're only eating 1 salad out per week!!

What do you do? **DO THE DIP!** You still want the taste –you still want the pleasure of eating your salad –right? Put your salad dressing on the side, dip your fork in the dressing and eat. It's that simple. You still get the same taste. You will cut out 95 % of those unwanted calories and still enjoy your meal. You can do this with any type of sauce or gravy. Bon Appetite!

Live Lean –Stay Lean

If you want less fat on you –you have to put less fat in you. Did you know that fat has double the amount of calories as Protein and Carbs? Let's look at the following chart.

Fat   9 calories per one gram
Protein   4 calories per one gram
Carbs   4 calories per one gram

As you can see, when you choose to eat high fat foods, the amount of calories that you ingest are significantly more than if you choose a healthier dose of complex carbs or lean protein.

Let's face it, fats are added to foods –because they make the food taste better. But, watch out for the little extra weight that follows!!

FOOD FOR THOUGHT: Replace 4 Tbsp of regular salad dressing with fat free vinaigrette and weigh 10 pounds less in one year.

Here are some healthy alternatives that will make your favorites a little less fatty. Personalize your modifications but always remember that the secret to success is *small* changes.

Recipe Calls:	Try This Instead:
1 egg	2 egg whites or ¼ egg substitute
Whole milk	1. 1 % milk 2. Skim milk
Mayonnaise	1. Lite mayonnaise 2. Fat-Free mayonnaise
Salad dressing	1. Reduced fat dressing 2. Fat-Free dressing or vinaigrette

Sour cream	1. Reduced fat sour cream
	2. Fat-Free sour cream or plain yogurt
Oil in baked goods	1. ½ oil and ½ fruit puree
	2. Fruit puree in equal amounts
Browning meat in oil	Use non-stick pan coated with nonfat vegetable spray
Fat for "greasing" the pan	Use nonfat vegetable spray
Sautéing vegetables in fat	1. Use ½ the fat called for and the remaining water
	2. Use all water
Cream	1. Reduced fat cream
	2. Evaporated skim milk
Broiling or steaming with fat	Sprinkle Butter Buds, Molly McButter or use spray margarine
Cheese	1. Reduced fat cheese Fat-Free cheese

Use mustard instead of mayonnaise. The "extras" can add on the calories and fat. A tablespoon of mayo will add on an extra 57 calories. How about another 106 calories for a single slice of cheese! Remember how many years it has taken to develop your taste buds…be patient in establishing new ones!

FOOD FOR THOUGHT: Substitute mustard or ketchup for mayo and weigh 10 pounds less in one year.

<u>**Helpful hint:**</u> Take a napkin and blot the oil off a pizza slice. This will lessen the amount of oil (which is 100 % fat) that you're consuming. You still get the taste—so why not do it?

"Put some bread with that butter." When you put a spread on your bread, make sure it goes on light. You just want the taste of the spread—it doesn't need to be slathered on. I like to watch people at restaurants just keep piling on the butter –I need you to become more aware of your "buttering" habits.

If you frequently challenge the chefs at finer restaurants, be forewarned that it is not uncommon to ingest an entire stick of butter before the meal is completed. In our terms, that's over 800 calories and 88 grams of fat!! You have to ask yourself the question…What's more important to you…. taste or a healthy heart?

Cut Fat – Not Favorites: Fat is essential to keeping your body functioning properly. <u>Adults need a minimum daily intake of 15 –25 grams per day</u> to ensure an adequate supply of essential fatty acids (EFA). These EFA's help our bodies develop, keep our skin healthy, keep our blood, arteries and nerves functioning properly and keep our metabolism running smoothly. As you'll notice, my plan incorporates a low fat approach to weight management, meaning low total fat. However, I do promote the majority of this fat coming from healthy fats such as polyunsaturated and monounsaturated fat.

I believe in eating foods rich in polyunsaturated and monounsaturated oils while limiting your saturated fat and trans fat intake. Saturated fats and trans fats are both major causes of high blood cholesterol levels –so beware.

Types of Polyunsaturated Fats

Nuts: walnuts

Plants

Seeds

Soybeans

Many types of fish

Healthy FAT = Monounsaturated Fat

Olive oil

Peanut oil

Canola oil

Avocado

Olives

Nuts: almonds, cashews, peanuts, pecans

Peanut butter

Sesame seeds

These fats have known to reduce blood cholesterol without reducing the protective cholesterol, HDL. Eat up! It has been documented that this healthy fat can lower your heart-disease risk. Stock your house with "good" fats: nuts, olive oil, avocados, fish, and soy.

**When I eat my salads at home, I sprinkle a small handful of nuts over salads. I also like to throw in a handful over pasta dishes and sometimes desserts. Beware –these are very easy to OVEREAT

**When you sauté, use 1-2 tablespoons of olive, peanut, sesame or canola oil. The aroma alone is worth the healthy calories

** When baking, use canola oil instead of butter or shortening. Any chance you get to help your heart with no additional calorie cost –do so!

** Use olive oil with balsamic vinegar –for a tasty, healthy full-fat salad dressing. Throw in a packet of Good Seasoning Italian dressing and you'll think you're in a fancy restaurant. Indulge yourself

**At our house, we love to dip bread into olive oil. 1 Tbsp of Olive oil has only 1.8 grams of saturated fat and 10 grams of healthy monounsaturated fat

**We also buy one or two Avocados per week and cut them into our salads. 1 Tbsp of Avocado less than 1 gram saturated fat and 2 grams of monounsaturated fat. Avocados also compliment with any salsa –Muy bueno!!

The Hoax of Hydrogenation

Both of these unsaturated fats can be turned into a saturated fat by a process called <u>hydrogenation</u> – adding hydrogen increases the stability of the oil, so it's usability improves for processing foods like baked goods and creamers. It also makes an unsaturated oil become more solid such as in the case of margarine. So, read your labels, and beware when you see the words "hydrogenated" or "partially hydrogenated." This process of hydrogenation is what produces <u>trans fats.</u>

Types of Saturated Fats

All Meats/All Dairies

Cheese

Egg yolks

Butter

Cream

How are solid fats different from oils?

Solid fats contain more **saturated fats** and/or *trans* **fats** than oils. Look for foods that are low in saturated fats, *trans* fats and cholesterol, to help reduce your risk of heart disease. *Trans* fats can be found in many cakes, cookies, crackers, icings, margarines, and microwave popcorns. Foods containing partially hydrogenated vegetable oils usually contain *trans* fats.

Solid fats are fats that are solid at room temperature, like butter and shortening. Solid fats come from many animal foods and like previously mentioned, can be made from vegetable oils through a process called hydrogenation. Some common solid fats are:

* Butter

* Beef fat (tallow, suet)

* Chicken fat

- Pork fat (lard)

- Stick margarine

- Shortening

Saturated fats, *trans* fats, and cholesterol tend to raise "bad" (LDL) cholesterol levels in the blood, which in turn increases the risk for heart disease. To lower risk for heart disease, cut back on foods containing saturated fats, *trans* fats and cholesterol.

Foods that are mainly oil include mayonnaise, most salad dressings, and soft (tub or squeeze) margarine with no *trans* fats. Check the Nutrition Facts label to find margarines with 0 grams of *trans* fat.

A few plant oils, however, including coconut oil and palm kernel oil, are high in saturated fats and for nutritional purposes should be considered to be solid fats.

FOOD FOR THOUGHT: Make most of your meals in a non-stick pan-and you'll automatically save 100 calories every time by eliminating the butter, margarine or oil used to grease the pan. Squirt a little non-stick cooking spray on the pan to manage your weight.

Goodbye to Fry

I highly recommend that you don't deep fry meats because this adds a significant amount of fat with no additional portion of food to nibble on.

The days of eating fried chicken wings on Monday nights must be evaluated. Suppose you had left 2 wings uneaten on your plate each week over the last decade. Significant? I'd say so… you'd save 30 pounds of body fat…. that's significant!

Chicken Breast without skin –
ROASTED   142 calories   3 grams of fat   19 % fat

Chicken Breast with skin -
FRIED   218 calories   8.7 grams of fat   36 % fat

This example shows you a whopping two and a half times more fat grams when the skin is on the meat and it's fried.

One way to eliminate some of the fat is to take off some or all of the breading and just eat the meat. You'll save yourself a tremendous amount of calories over time and still enjoy the flavor. Alternatively, eat a smaller portion of the fried meal or really watch the frequency in which you indulge.

FILL UP – TRIM DOWN!

Numbers Game

When it comes to calories and energy balance, this is one big, gigantic numbers game. As we discussed, 3500 calories equals one pound of fat. Can't get around this figure. I've given you a few selections to show you that any extra calories coming in on a daily basis that don't get burned off –make a huge difference on the scale in the course of one year.

One Extra Per day	Pounds gained after one year
2 tbsp of Salad dressing (250 cal)	26 pounds
20. Ounce Regular pop (200)	25 pounds
2 lite Beers (200 cal)	21 pounds
1 grand latte (160 cal)	17 pounds
½ cup Light Ice Cream (120 cal)	12.5 pounds
½ cup of Cereal (95 cal)	10 pounds
3.5 ounces of Wine (70 cal)	7 pounds

Healthy Cooking Methods: You want to get the most nutritional value out of all your food. For healthiest results, cook your foods thoroughly – but RAPIDLY. You want to get lean and stay lean --I recommend grilling, broiling, roasting, stewing, poaching, pressure cooking, steaming, stir frying and baking for the majority of your meal preparations.

"Ahead of you are new challenges and goals. They may seem mere shadows today, but they will one day be central to your life. It seems such a paradox to look backward and forward at once, but the significance of any achievement exists in that very contradiction. Without your past, you have nothing on which to build your future. Without the future, your past would have no opportunity to come into full bloom."

--Anonymous

Day 11
DAILY VICTORIES QUICK FIX: Fiber Up

"Whatever you paint in your mind, the mind goes to work to complete"
- Anonymous

Fiber fills you up...not out. I'm going to go out on the limb and make a safe assumption to say, that if you're currently not eating a diet consisting of plenty of fruits, vegetables and whole grains, that you're probably not getting the **20-35 grams of daily fiber** recommended by both the American Heart Association and the American Institute for Cancer Research. The average American eats **only about 11 grams** of fiber daily.

When you follow my **GET LEAN IN 15** menus, you'll mainly stick to fiber-rich complex carbohydrates. You'll be energized without the feeling of that metabolic roller coaster ride. Fiber helps stabilize blood sugar by blocking absorption sites of sugar, so less will be absorbed into the blood stream and at a slower pace.

Whenever you have a choice between whole grain and regular enriched wheat/white products, I advise **ALWAYS** to choose the whole grain item to ensure a higher fiber count. The extra fiber will accentuate the feeling of fullness that, in turn, will help your weight loss efforts. Fiber makes you absorb fewer calories. For every one-gram of fiber that you consume, you absorb approximately seven fewer calories from food.

The insoluble fiber found in whole grain breads and cereals, and many fruits and vegetables binds with water to help waste move out of the body smoothly. A high fiber diet reduces the risk of gastrointestinal cancers by maintaining bowel regularity. This may be an odd request.... but, I need you to have healthy, regular bowel movements –quit snickering. Not only is this healthy for you, but becoming regular makes you feel less "bloaty" which makes a difference in your weight control plan - psychologically.

It also helps prevent the re-absorption of cholesterol into the blood stream by pulling it out of the body. Keep in mind, that as you begin to increase your fiber intake, it's important to <u>increase your water </u>intake to keep it moving through your body. Fiber acts like a sponge. It will absorb the water, adding bulk to your stool, making it softer and easier to eliminate from the body.

Fiber for your Figure. Make an effort to eat raw, crunchy vegetables, for a smart and filling snack. You really can't eat too much of the crunchy stuff!

Crunchy vegetables are so full of fiber and water that a full cup of green beans, for example, has less than 40 calories. Snack on raw carrots, celery, radishes, mushrooms, spinach and broccoli.

As I discussed earlier, I like to put my vegetables covered, in the microwave, and cook for a few minutes, and then sprinkle with just a little bit of butter granules (zero calories) or serve with tomato salsa. Eat as much as you like of raw or slightly steamed, crunchy vegetables.

Here's a list of high fiber foods. I recommend making just one or two changes in your daily habits that can really push you toward a respectable dose of fiber.

FIBER   7 grams or more
100% Bran Cereal 1/2 cup
Butter beans 1/2 cup
Fiber One Cereal 1/2 cup
Navy beans 1/2 cup
Kidney beans 1/2cup

FIBER 5-6 grams
Peas 1/2 cup
Raisin Bran Cereal 3/4 cup
Black beans 1/2 cup
Bran Flakes 3/4 cup
Brussels sprouts 1/2 cup
Lentils 1/2 cup

FIBER 2-4 grams
Prunes, dried 4
Oatmeal 3/4 cup
Popcorn 3 cups
Potato 1 small
Pears 1/2 large
Pumpernickel bread 1 slice
Apple 1 (include the skin with your fruit)
Apricots 4
Broccoli 1/2 cup
Green Beans 1/2 cup
Strawberries 1 cup
Carrots 1

My wife brought this mix to our marriage. Mix three or more different cans of beans and some diet Italian dressing. Eat this three-bean salad all week. It's quick, tasty, and healthy.

Pantry Patrol. Replace white flour grains with whole wheat grains, and you can expect to double your fiber intake. Remember to drink LOTS of water!! Look for the first ingredient on the food label to be "whole wheat" or "whole grain."

- 100 % Whole Grain Bread

- Whole Wheat Pancakes or Waffles

- Whole Wheat Pita or Buns

- Whole Grain Crackers

- Brown Rice

- Brown Pasta

- Higher Fiber Cereals/whole grain cereals

  (> 5 grams fiber per serving)

- Oatmeal

- Dry Peas, Lentils, Beans

Do you eat whole grain bread? Almost everyone says yes to that question. But the fact is many of you would be surprised to learn that your bread might not be whole wheat or whole grain. It's legal for the package to say 'wheat bread' on the label, but not have any whole wheat in the ingredient list. The label is a marketing program. ……And the ingredient list is the <u>facts!</u>

All wheat flour is wheat. So it can be wheat flour, but not be whole wheat. The first ingredient in whole wheat bread must be whole wheat flour. If it says flour, enriched wheat, wheat flour or any other word choices other than whole wheat flour then it is not whole wheat.

A Dietitian's Dream Day. I asked our Dietitian, Kim Tessmer, to give us an example of what type of tips she would recommend to one of her clients in a personal setting. You'll be surprised to note that most of her helpful hints are in alignment with the GET LEAN IN 15 plan.

Eat breakfast each and everyday! Whatever you can fit in! A bowl of whole grain cereal, fat-free milk and fruit is quick and easy and starts your day out right!

Take a piece of fruit to work with you everyday to eat as a snack or with lunch. Once you accomplish this goal—increase to two fruits. And stick to a variety of fruits.

Start at least one meal a day with a fresh salad. For convenience at home or at work, buy pre-cut, packaged salad ingredients that can be assembled in no time. Top it with a variety of raw vegetables and a low fat salad dressing.

Display several different fresh fruits in a bowl on your table at home. Eat one fruit from the bowl every day.

Besides being packed full of nutrients, fruits and vegetables can also be quite filling. They may even ward off any empty calorie snacking that might follow! Don't be discouraged by the recommended 5 to 9 servings a day. The guide below shows that one serving is less than what you might think.

One serving equals:

1 medium piece of fruit

½ grapefruit

½ cup fruit or vegetables (raw, cooked, canned, or frozen)

1 cup of leafy salad greens

¼ cup of dried fruit

¾ cup or 6 oz. of 100% juice

½ cup cooked peas or beans

1 medium potato

Combine fruit with your main meal courses. Raisins, apples and tangerine slices add sweet, crunchy variety to a salad. Apples complement pork, pineapple is great with fish, and orange slices are perfect with chicken.

Never miss snack time –eating small meals throughout the day prevents hunger and keeps metabolism high- just be sure to choose healthier snacks and remember, this is a snack-NOT a meal!

Eat small amounts of healthy fats and lean protein at every meal to create a feeling of fullness.

Switch to "whole" grain or "whole" wheat breads as well as brown rice instead of white. The extra fiber and added nutrients help to promote good health!

Make it a habit to drink at least one, preferably two glasses of fat free milk every day or choose low-fat yogurt.

Use a smaller dinner plate so you are not tempted to eat more than you really need.

Though these are just a few tips that Kim might start you off with, take heed of her suggestions! She charges over a $ 100 an hour to give the same advice.

Day 12
DAILY VICTORIES QUICK FIX: Weigh to Goal

"Wise living consists perhaps less in acquiring good habits than in acquiring as few habits as possible"
- Anonymous

A GOAL is more than a dream. It's a dream being acted upon. Success in life is not about a matter of inches or pounds …it's taking the first steps towards a reachable GOAL.

If your personal GOAL is <u>finally</u> to lose the weight and **KEEP** it off --- my combination of Portion Control and Gentle Movement is a proven formula that lets you eat the foods you **LOVE** and keeps you healthy by increasing activity that fits your busy lifestyle. The most important thing to realize is that it's <u>not</u> where you were …or where you are, but WHERE YOU WANT TO GET TO!

You must form an image **NOW** of the person you want to be at GOAL weight. When you get obsessed about a personal GOAL – you receive energy, physical power and enthusiasm needed to accomplish your GOAL ----you will have AUTOMATIC SELF MOTION, which enables you to make healthy lifestyle choices on a regular basis –WITHOUT EVEN THINKING ABOUT IT!

<u>**Suggested GOALS.**</u> It's important to have SPECIFIC goals that you can calculate. Here are a few examples that will help you determine your own goals and desires.

- Lose 10 % of my body weight
- Stay at the same size, but firm my entire lower body
- Start enjoying tennis, golf, dancing _____ etc.…
- Get a firmer, rounded buns area
- Tighten my abs –fit into my old jeans

- Feel better about what I can't change and change the things I can
- Have more energy and motivation to move more
- Work on balancing out my diet and including all the food groups each day
- Build my arm strength

Be nice to yourself—We are all <u>IMPERFECT BODIES!!</u> Yep that's right-I said it. The pressure's off. You, me and everyone you know…. we are all <u>just average</u>-all our bodies have strengths and weaknesses. We are unique, individual special selves. Hey, I wish I were taller. Too bad, that's not reality–so I do my best with what God gave me to work with.

There are certain things you can change, and other things that you have no control over and therefore, can't change. I will help you with the parts you do have control over and can change. But, don't have unrealistic expectations when you start a weight management plan. Make your goals SPECIFIC and REALISTIC!

10 % of your body weight!!

A very realistic, short-term goal would be to FOCUS on losing ONLY 10 percent present body weight. I used this method with all my clients. It establishes a precedent for success. I know…barring a catastrophe, that my clients, as well as you, will lose 10 percent of your present body weight following my basic system. This gives you the motivation and confidence in the system to keep moving forward. Also, it doesn't feel like a never-ending journey to get to your long-term goal weight.

Example: If you weigh 150 pounds X 10 % = 15 pounds
150 – 15 pounds = **135 pounds –your first goal weight**

200 pounds X 10 % = 20 pounds
200 – 20 = **180 pounds-your first goal weight**

When you give yourself small GOALS – FAILURE IS IMPOSSIBLE!!

Creating a plan for lean living requires many steps. The first step is to know what your ultimate goal is. I've given you the blueprint for success in the menus and fitness plan. However, no one ever said that following a weight loss program would be easy. Over the years, I've found that sticking to your plan is easier when you have support and encouragement from your family and friends.

Don't be shy. You can get support from the closest people in your life –by asking them for it. Yes, that's right. Tell them that you're committed to being healthy and fit, and let them know that you need their help as well.

Your family and friends need to:

- Appreciate your efforts
- Encourage you to continue no matter what obstacles come your way
- Give you time for yourself –especially when it comes to your exercise plan
- It's your time to exercise –NO ONE GETS IT!
- Give you constant positive feedback

It helps to have people to talk to when you're having problems with your diet and exercise program. Your family and friends can help you by:

- Listening to problems you are having sticking to your plan
- Letting you know they believe in you and admire what you're doing
- Reminding you of your commitment and the benefits you're experiencing

Don't Go It Alone. If you're like most people, you may need a little extra ounce of motivation to continue your quest. It makes perfectly good sense to get a "lean buddy." Ask a friend or family member to join you with your new lifestyle.

You and your partner will be your own support system. It tends to be more fun and easier to be enthusiastic about going for walks or doing a workout if you have someone to go with.

I know sometimes it's tough to stay consistent by yourself. Your "lean buddy" wont make you quit. There's a lot to say about accountability. If you know that you have someone that's counting on you, it's a natural instinct to try not to let that person down.

Here are a few tips when looking for that special lean buddy:

- Try motivating your spouse or partner to become that special one. There have been studies that have shown that married couples actually have more luck sticking to a program if they do it together. I've always told clients, "the couple that weighs together, stays together"

- Make sure your partner has goals similar to yours. Just because your friends with the lady at church, doesn't mean that she'll stay committed to your walking schedule

- You must have similar schedules. Remember, time is the biggest factor for an unhealthy lifestyle. So, this will be a built-in excuse if you are fighting the time issue from the beginning

- Make sure your buddy brings **PMA** to the table. That's **P**ositive **M**ental **A**ttitude. The last thing you want or need is a whiner or someone brings constant stress to the relationship. If a person were negative, I'd advise cutting the strings early on if you're to be consistent with your lifestyle journey

- Tell everyone you know that you're starting a weight management program. You may be surprised how many people are in the same frame of mind as you–but didn't know how to approach the subject. Ask around. You'll be able to reach out to plenty of potential "buddies"

DO IT NOW!

How do you make the secret of getting things done a part of your life.........by habit! Develop habits by repetition.

You are what your habits make you – YOU can choose your habits.

The secret to getting things done – is to ACT. Be a self-motivator – Do it now!

When you say *Do it now* – you need to react on it – just don't say it and don't do anything.

Do it now in little things. Don't procrastinate. That means if it's a phone call- call NOW, the alarm clock rings – get up NOW, you need to make a sale – go after customers NOW.

An old saying: SUCCESS MUST BE CONTINUALLY PRACTICED – OR IT WILL TAKE WINGS AND FLY AWAY!!   Now is the time to act.

The secret of getting things done can change a person's attitude from negative to positive. Now is the time –before it becomes "yesterday, I should have…" What prevents us from doing the things we want? Shyness in the face of our inspirations. Sometimes were afraid of our ideas – it takes a certain boldness to step out on an untested idea. Trust me I know, being an entrepreneur for the past 10 years, it's not easy, but with tenacity your dreams can be met. It's this kind of boldness that produces spectacular results.

SELF TALK –BE CAREFUL WHO'S LISTENING

We're all guilty of it. Negative self-talk. We can be our worst critics and harshest judges. We can do more damage with our thoughts than anyone else. We need to make a conscious effort to STOP it - before it STOPS you.

It's the voice in our head that says things like:

	THE ACTION YOU TAKE
• I can't do this	NONE
• It's not going to work	NONE
• I won't stick with it-I never do	NONE
• There's no way, it's too hard	NONE
• I'm too fat	NONE
• I hate my thighs	NONE
• I have a big butt	NONE
• I don't have any willpower	NONE

This type of self-talk is very self-defeating and probably comes from the idea of fear of failure. It's our defense mechanism that we develop to protect us from experiencing emotions or feelings we believe will be unpleasant. Stop the negative words before they come out.

What are the exact words you're telling yourself? Do you honestly desire to fail? Do you really believe you can't succeed?

When you break down these negative thoughts in these terms –you can see how self-destroying this becomes. You will progress with your plan quicker if that little voice doesn't rear its ugly head every time you want to do something good for yourself. Recognize negative self-talk –keep an "open" ear –it's usually charged with emotional energy–it will not be hard to miss.

Retrace your thoughts..........mentally retrace your steps and work your way back into thinking positive. Try to figure out what your feelings were before the negative words. Was it doubt? Was it guilt? Was it anxiety or frustration?

When you experience an unpleasant feeling or emotion…

- Take it for what it is

- Think about it

- Try to understand it

- And then **MOVE ON!!!**

Just because you may have had an emotional experience the last time you wanted to change an issue in your life — it doesn't mean you'll experience the same emotion this time!

So, let's see how this works in real life. You say to yourself "I can't do it, I'm just meant to be fat."

Retracing: "Wait a second, here I go again. What am I feeling right now? What caused this negative talk? The last time I tried to lose weight wasn't the best experience for me. I guess I'm anxious about getting my hopes up and then failing again. I felt so disappointed in myself last time. Guilty is a better word."

The **GET LEAN IN 15** rethinking plan: "Well, who says the same thing has to happen again. Right now, I want to make a change. I'm tired of feeling this way about myself. I know what I need to do and I believe I'm capable of doing it. I'm going to go forward, try my best, and take one day at a time. If I blow it, **it's no big deal;** I'll just keep trying. I'm not going to let my fears control me. I'm in this for the long run. THIS TIME WILL BE DIFFERENT!"

COMMIT ---EMBRACE THE CHALLENGE

MEDIA MISCONCEPTIONS

You've seen commercial products advertise on TV, Radio, Catalogs, and Magazine ads, Billboard ads----the media message is CLEAR:

- LOSE WEIGHT and BE SEXIER!
- LOSE WEIGHT and BE HAPPIER!
- LOSE WEIGHT, HAVE MORE FUN!
- LOSE WEIGHT, HAVE MORE FRIENDS!

What's the message here? Whatever you do. …DON'T GET FAT! Keep in mind, most of this is Hollywood fluff…these models are air brushed, and they don't represent a realistic standard. So, try not to compare. I know it's human nature to compare…however, you and I and everyone on this planet will always fail by comparison. There's always going to be someone better looking, better body, more financially fit, etc…you name it.

Remember this about YOU:

YOU are not "inferior"
YOU are not "superior"
YOU are simply "YOU"
YOU are not in competition with any other person simply because there is not another person on the face of the earth like YOU

YOU are an INDIVIDUAL
YOU are UNIQUE
YOU are not like any other person
YOU are not "supposed" to be like any other person and no other
person is "supposed" to be like you

Like who YOU are …right now. Your health depends on it

Food For Thought: <u>Faulty Perceptions or Reality?</u>

More than ever, women are dissatisfied with their weight and bodies. Thinness has become the yardstick for success or failure –a gauge that every woman can be measured. Instead of constantly worrying if your body is "measuring up," take some time and think about the things that make you feel good about yourself.

Visualize what you want yourself to look like. Take a look at your picture each day. Everyone's ideal self is different.

When you look in the mirror to check out how your thighs are shaping up –you may not be seeing yourself accurately. Try to draw your attention away from your problem part and take PRIDE in your whole body.

If you feel that you will fail no matter what –what do you think the outcome will BE? With just a little change in attitude - You can find good in any situation. The beauty of this is that YOU have complete control. You can change your self image-You are the director of your own movie. Those "big hips" have now become "not bad" for someone who works as hard as you do, or has 3 kids, etc…You're doing the BEST you can do for yourself at the present moment. You need to find a realistic view of yourself. Somebody you're comfortable with—you're creating a new YOU.

Someone you can trust and believe.

Someone you can be proud of.

Someone who has unlimited self-confidence.

Someone who has a positive self-outlook on himself and others.

FOOD FOR THOUGHT: What you believe determines your relationships...not just with others – but also with YOURSELF.

HOPE is the magic ingredient in setting goals. It can best be described as aspiration with the expectation of obtaining what is desired and belief that it is attainable.

1. Desirable
2. Believable
3. Attainable

Greatness comes to those who develop a BURNING DESIRE to achieve high goals. DREAM BIG !!

Success is achieved and maintained by those who try and keep on trying-no matter what gets in their way.

To become an ACHIEVER in anything-you need to PRACTICE, PRACTICE, and PRACTICE!

BRAND NEW ME

Day 13
DAILY VICTORIES QUICK FIX: Empty Your Calories

"I can give you a six word formula for success; think things through-then follow through"
- Edward Rickenbacker

EC's –empty calories. We love them, but they don't love us. This may be harsh, but if you want a sure way to remain at your present weight- choose empty calorie snacks over healthier choices and **I guarantee** that you'll be doomed into diet failure for eternity. You might think that an *empty calorie* refers to a food that is low in calories. However, these types of food choices offer little or no nutritional value. For example, a nutrition bar and a candy bar may have the same number of calories, but where the nutritional bar contains fiber and some vitamins and minerals essential to good nutrition, the candy bar may be completely comprised of sugar. Hence, the name –empty calories. I recommend that you practice moderation and control by giving yourself **a limit of 3–5 times per week** and pre-plan as often as possible. Your action plan is to **eliminate one "Empty Calorie" food everyday (EC).**

What are <u>examples</u> of EC's?

- Regular soft drinks

- Candy

- Cakes

- Cookies

- Pies

- Fruit drinks, such as fruitades and fruit punch

- Milk-based desserts and products, such as ice cream, sweetened yogurt and sweetened milk

- Grain products such as sweet rolls and cinnamon toast

I'm not saying completely cut these foods from your eating habits, because I feel that's unrealistic. Special occasion foods, snacks and beverages are a part of any practical and healthy lifestyle. However, these foods provide lots of empty calories with very little nutritional value. Sharp label reading skills are a must to work in your favorite snacks!

First, read the serving size at the top of the label. Second, read the calories per serving. Know how much you're eating and how many calories that serving size will add to your day. You can always adjust the serving size to keep the calories where you want them. The following list gives you **examples of 100-200 calorie items** that can be worked into the day instead of adding on any additional calories for the day.

½ cup ice cream or sherbet

¾ cup low fat or sugar free ice cream

1/8 single crusted, fruit or custard pie

2 fun sized candy bars

6 Hershey Kisses

¼ cup mixed nuts

2 –2 1/2 " diameter cookies

handful of snack chips

2 ½" x 2 ½ cube of frosted cake

1 granola bar

1 – ¾" x ¾" inch cube of cheese

1 small doughnut/plain cake

3 cups non-air popped popcorn

8-12 crackers

6 cups air popped popcorn

Keep in mind, when you eat snacks they usually take the place of a healthier food choice. The calories are still counted and added to your daily total. So, when snacks are eaten, you're going to have to eliminate another food to accommodate the extra calories coming in from the snack. With your pre-planned **GET LEAN IN 15** menus, snacks are already a part of your calorie intake! With a little pre-planning, snacks can fit in with no problem!

We all snack…and that's a perfectly healthy way of eating. I want to show you some great tips on snacking light –snacking right.

 FOOD FOR THOUGHT: Afternoon delight! If you're hungry in the afternoon -- even if it's close to dinner -- eat something! Do it now. Approaching dinner in a ravenous state is asking for a binge. It's especially important to eat an afternoon snack if dinner is late. *Bottom line: A planned snack can save you at least 300 calories a night*

Stock up on healthy, portable snacks

When you're grocery shopping, pick up bags of baby carrots, string cheese, nuts, fresh and dried fruit, single serving packs of applesauce, yogurt, whole grain crackers, peanut butter, turkey jerky, etc…. Having healthy portable snacks around will help you avoid unhealthy vending machine, convenience store and fast-food options.

 FOOD FOR THOUGHT: Total Control! Get rid of the foods in your house that you have a problem controlling. Bottom line: If that saves just one 500-calorie binge per week, you could lose 7 pounds in a year.

Chips and other hand picking snacks can be a deceivingly sneaky way to not fill you up…but fill you out. Store bought tortilla chips may seem like a good option when quickly glancing over the food label. However, upon close inspection, you'll see that while the calorie count may seem low (140 calories per serving), the serving size is only 11 chips –who can stop there? Typical mindless munching in front of the TV can make you take in far more calories than you realized. With this in mind, look carefully at the serving size and servings per container, not just the calories listed per serving, when reading packages food labels.

Any food item that passes your lips has the potential to turn to fat if you're taking in more than you're burning off in any given day. Take the extra time to look carefully at food labels and be aware of portion sizes. Reaching a goal does mean changing your lifestyle, but that change doesn't have to be painful.

FOOD FOR THOUGHT: More snacking, fewer calories! People who snack between meals find it easier to lose weight because they actually take in fewer calories. Snacks keep you satisfied so you're less likely to experience runaway hunger or emotional cravings. Snacks have to be planned. Otherwise, you'll find yourself stuck with whatever's available. *Bottom line: If your healthy snack keeps you from your usual vending machine pick-me-up, you'll save about 250 calories right there. Do it every day and you'll lose a lot of weight in a hurry.*

Moderate don't Eliminate. If you restrict yourself from eating all added sugar, you may focus on the deprivation of your sweet tooth and fuel a sugar binge. Portion sizes are getting larger in this category of simple sugars – which is part of the problem- so be smart and split your chocolate cake or apple pie alamode. P.S. Sometimes a little sugar is good for your soul.

SIMPLE vs. COMPLEX

There is a huge difference between simple sugars and complex sugars. A few years ago, carbs were given a bad name. "I can't have any carbs" use to be the mantra for millions. However, all carbs were not created equal. This is a quick intro to Carbs 101…

Simple (EC's) Empty Calories!! - White table sugar, white flour, cakes, cookies, candy, and other desserts

Complex –whole grains, vegetables, cereals, beans

What happens when your car's gas tank is on empty? You stall. The same is true about your body in relation to carbohydrate intake – Without carbohydrates – you run out of gas. Your body begins to burn what's called a ketone body, the bi-product of fat metabolism. In fact, if you make a habit of eating low carbohydrates, you could get bad breath, feel weak and lightheaded, lose some hair, and risk damaging your heart- that's no fun!

Simple carbs are empty calorie types of foods (except for fruit) and have very little nutritional value. They can only do one thing – run your daily calorie count up and make you overweight. The "rush" you feel when eating these simple sugars is due to the rapid rise in blood sugar that they cause.   Yet remember, "What goes up must come down."   And when your blood sugar drops abruptly, you feel lethargic and wiped out. I'm sure you've experienced this reaction-it's quite noticeable.

When you experience this roller coaster feeling, what do you look for almost instinctively to counteract the low? Let me guess, a candy bar or a can of pop? We crave sugar. The USDA says that the average American consumes <u>20 teaspoons of added sugar a day </u>-that's incredible, because that represents 16 – 20 % of total daily caloric intake.

These empty calories can do only one thing – put on weight. And if you're getting this many calories in your diet from these empty calories, it doesn't leave a lot of room for balanced, wholesome, healthy, nutrient dense foods. People who are overweight can still be undernourished. Eating more healthful foods is a good way to improve your health and lower your calorie intake at the same time.

The USDA recommends that adults get no more than 6-10 percent of their daily calories from added sugar (approximately 6 teaspoons per 1600 calories). Added sugars are sugars and syrups that are added to foods or beverages during processing or preparation. This does not include naturally occurring sugars such as those that occur in milk and fruits.

A SPOONFUL OF SUGAR…………………….….

Foods	Teaspoons of Sugar
Pop (8oz)	6
Chocolate cake with icing (1/6 of 9 inch sq.)	10
Ice Cream Sundae (2 scoops ice cream, 2 Tbsp syrup)	7
Fruit cocktail (1/2 cup)	5

Fructose sounds like fruit- so it must be healthy?

High-fructose corn syrup, an added sweetener, is the worst sugar there is, and it can be found in countless foods and beverages. High fructose corn syrup has been linked to obesity and type 2 diabetes.

Some researchers believe that high fructose corn syrup actually acts like a fat in the body more than sugar and that it may trigger mechanisms that promote body-fat storage. However, more research still needs to be done to prove these theories. In any case, read your food labels and look for this little sugar sneak!

It seems these days; the magical number for keeping your sweet tooth in check is to **stay under 100 calories** for the sweet. This list should help you decide the serving size to stay under.

25 M&M's

15 Jellybeans

Two handfuls of Chocolate Raisins

1/2 an apple spread with 2 tsp. peanut butter

2 inch slice Sponge cake

1 Banana

½ cup Non-Fat fruit yogurt

½ cup Sherbet

Single serving Fat-Free pudding cup

Dole Fruit bar

Whole wheat toast with 1 tsp. sugar-free spread

Single serving of Apple Sauce

Day 14
DAILY VICTORIES QUICK FIX: Get Fruity

"An obstacle is something you see when you take your eyes off your goal"
- Anonymous

Notice your menus that Kim, the RD, has provided. Every day the menus contain at least 2 servings of fruit. I want to point out how easy it is to fit them into your routine. Like vegetables, fruits are power packed with nutrients, as well as fiber and they help to add to your feeling of fullness.

You will notice the more fruits you eat –the thinner you feel. It may be a placebo effect (thinking that something will help you)--but I find it very difficult after I eat a granny smith apple, to feel anything but leaner. By the way, it's hard to over consume too much fruit –when's the last time you gobbled down two apples rapidly? It's difficult, because of the fiber content. However, even fruit has calories so don't over-do it and keep within your calorie range.

To be successful, you need to manage your hunger. I need you to make a serious effort to follow this guideline of **adding a minimum of 2 fruits every day.** As you know, choosing to include more fruits and vegetables is a big leap towards a healthier diet. The "5 A Day " plan would like for you to eat at least 5 servings of fruits and vegetables every day.

These foods will not only help reduce your risk for some forms of cancer and for heart disease, fruits and vegetables are waistline friendly. Fruits help you become leaner because you fill up on this wholesome choice and end up eating less of other foods.

By the way, nobody is telling you to give up meat and become a vegetarian. Despite the known health benefits of fruits and vegetables, too few

Americans are eating the recommended amounts of these foods. A new study finds that just 17 percent of women aged 51 to 70 meet their fruity goal, and among other age groups, nearly 90 percent are falling short.

But be careful – one medium orange has approximately 60 calories, while an 8 ounce glass of OJ has about 110 calories (and no fiber).

In trying to stay with the American Diabetes Association recommendations, I strongly encourage eating fruit rather than drinking down the calories as juice. The closer to nature you are with your selection, the more fiber and nutrients you'll gain. In perspective, an orange is better than orange juice, which is better than an orange fruit roll-up!! Add fruit's low-fat fiber, flavor and bulk to baked goods, smoothies and salads.

FOOD FOR THOUGHT: Fruit to the Rescue! People who eat 5 pieces of fruit per day have a 38 percent lower risk of stroke than those eating less fruit.

Fresh vs. Frozen/Canned

There have been studies showing that many canned fruits and vegetables have as much nutritional value as eating these foods fresh. Also, frozen foods can make an excellent substitute for fresh produce. Canned and frozen fruits and vegetables are picked when fully ripe and nutrients are at their peak. The immediate processing preserves the natural nutrient value.

On the other hand, fresh produce is sometimes picked when it's under ripe which could compromise its value. It usually takes several days for fresh produce to get to you,-the consumer, and so more nutrients are lost.

When you choose canned fruits, avoid those packed in heavy syrup. The syrup is simple sugar that, again, will increase the calories without increasing the nutritional value.

The bottom line…. life is hectic, so whatever way you can **eat your 2 fruits every day** – whether it be fresh, dried, frozen or canned - eating your fruits is what's paramount. Convenience to your lifestyle will dictate your success!

Some FRUITY choices...

Apricots	Papaya
Passion fruit	Bananas
Pear	Blackberries
Pineapple	Cantaloupe
Plum	Cherries
Raspberries	Grapefruit
Star fruit	Honeydew
Strawberries	Kiwi
Tangerine	Orange
Watermelon	

More Exotic choices of fruits...

Asian Pears	Quinces
Clementines	Passion Fruit
Pomegranates	Mango

Day 15
DAILY VICTORIES QUICK FIX: One Meal at a Time

"If you think you can win, you can win. Faith is necessary to Victory"
-William Hazlit

This is a mantra that I have my clients follow every day. To achieve <u>Maximum Success</u> ---Progress is made **One Meal** at a time.

Instead of trying to reach your ultimate goal – which is <u>never</u> gaining unwanted weight again, try to make a HEALTHIER choice each meal. You have approximately 35 opportunities during each week (3 meals + 2 snacks X 7 days) to make a healthy choice. You don't have to be perfect. In fact, if you can choose a healthy choice 80 percent of the time or 28 meals ... you **will** reach your GOAL. Commit this question to your mind on everything you eat ...*Will this help me get to where I want to go??*

ONE MEAL AT A TIME

Meal by Meal
Day by Day
Week by Week
Month by Month
Year by Year

Learn It!!   Live It!!   Lose It!!   Love It!!

As if it's not already, eating out is about to become a bigger and bigger dieting challenge. Sticking to your guns away from home is hard for many reasons. They all seem to boil down to this dilemma: How can you possibly have control of your diet when you don't control your eating environment? But, here's the surprise—you CAN control your environment, no matter where you eat! It's important to know that you're the customer and you're in charge.

We spend more money and waste more calories by dining out than ever before. The National Restaurant Association estimates that we eat almost six meals per week outside the home (about 290 times per year) -- which means it's important to know how to eat out and still live a lean lifestyle.

The National Restaurant Association says that these meals take up 44 percent of our food budgets. This could grow to 53 percent in the next few years. You don't have to bust your calorie budget every time you eat away from your home. Here are some ideas and strategies that will help you take charge of your next culinary adventure, every step of the way:

- You don't have to do a complete 360 (degrees) to eat lean. Just a few small changes in the way you order can make a drastic difference. First, remember that restaurants are in business to serve their customers, and most restaurants will make sure you get what you want. They want to have repeat customers. So, don't be afraid to ask questions and demand the type of food that makes your new lifestyle tasty and healthy

- You should NOT feel embarrassed. You're the only one who will be in agony. Tell the server that you're allergic to certain foods or that you have certain medical conditions so you can't eat the food prepared an unhealthy way

- You will begin to take pride in the fact that you will master every restaurant that you go in. Bottom line…get what you want!!

- But even cutting a mere 100 calories every time you eat (3 meals a day) can result in losing more than 31 pounds in one year (365 x 300 calories = 109,500 calories, divided by 3,500 calories (1 pound of fat) =31 pounds in one year

It's easy to cut out 100 calories at your table:

*Instead of sour cream and/or butter on your baked potato, try salsa
*Do without a piece of bread or a roll with margarine at meals
*Remove the skin from chicken before or after cooking

- Instead of full fat mayo for sandwiches or tuna salad use a small amount of light mayo or plain yogurt
- Replace cheese with tomatoes, lettuce, onions on your sandwich or hamburger
- Replace your favorite soft drink with a glass of ice cold water
- Leave 3-4 bites of food on your plate at each meal and don't go for seconds
- Instead of fruit juice choose a piece of fruit, which will cut calories and fill you up more
- Grab a handful of your favorite snack and put the bag away!
- Substitute a no-calorie sweetener for sugar in each cup of coffee you drink daily
- Use a non-stick skillet or cooking spray instead of butter when stove-top cooking
- Choose tuna packed in water instead of tuna packed in oil
- Use light or fat-free dressing on your salads instead of the regular version and leave off the croutons
- Reduce your portion of pasta and or rice by ½ cup
- Choose thin crust pizza as opposed to thick crust
- Top your pizza with vegetables and leave off the fatty meats such as sausage and pepperoni as well as double cheese
- Stick to one cup of cereal and fill the rest of the bowl with fresh fruit
- Spread all-fruit spread on your morning toast instead of butter or margarine
- Grill a vegetable burger or turkey burger instead of a beef burger
- Replace your breaded fish sticks with grilled fresh fish
- Replace your daily candy bar with a piece of fresh fruit
- Swap full fat salad dressing for the reduced fat version

Most restaurants these days have a computer presence. If I have any doubt of what healthy choices are on the menu, I usually check out their menu on the website or I just call and check out the healthier selections. When all else fails, I usually improvise with the menus at most restaurants. I can order a lean protein selection –chicken or fish, and tell them to put the meat on top of a salad- healthy and quick!

One of the sure giveaways for an unhealthier choice is if the selection is fried. I always ask if the food is fried. You can ask them to grill it or bake it to lower the calories. The cost stays the same –so, there's no harm to the restaurant by cooking it this way.

I also ask what type of sauce is on top of the food. I try to stay away from white sauces; creams, dressings, gravies. Anything white usually means it's made from cream and is loaded with fat. Or, just ask to put the sauce on the side. Look out for those cheese sauces. Again........loaded with fat. If you still have to order with the cheese –just pull some of the cheese off the top of the food. It will save you those unwanted saturated fat calories.

I always ask my server to show me by hand length how big the serving size is. It's very easy to see if the meat is going to fit in the palm of your hand or if it's going to be the size of a football.

Ask the server to not put extra salt on the food. And I'd advise you not to pick up the salt shaker on your table and start shakin'. I will tell you adding salt does not have any calories in it or fat-and therefore, will not harm your weight loss plan- however, it does increase your chances to elevate your blood pressure.

Restaurant savvy

If you're like most of us, you probably eat out quite a few times during the week. Here are a few hints on how to win this war at the dinner table.

Split the entrée in half and ask for a side salad. If alone, ask for the entrée to be divided in half and packaged in a carryout before it comes to the table. Gain an edge on hunger by starting with a broth based soup, fruit, raw vegetables, or a light seafood appetizer.

Instead of having a main meal- it's OK to order 2 healthy appetizers in one sitting. This can provide a healthy advantage as the portions are smaller and you have a variety of nutritious choices. Don't stuff yourself – as your stomach expands –so does your appetite!

Keep good company. Talking more and eating less will ensure that you'll enjoy your meal without overindulging.

If you're going to have a piece of bread before the meal, (which is perfectly fine by the way) then I would advise not to order something that is "bready" like a sandwich or pizza.

"Not as healthy" preparation words….any food described as buttery, breaded, buttered, fried, pan-fried, creamed, scalloped, au gratin, a la mode.

Healthy preparation words ….any food described as grilled, baked, steamed, broiled, poached, stir-fried, roasted or blackened.

Avoid sauces made with milk, cheese, oil or mayonnaise. Marinara and tomato-based sauces are usually more flavorful and healthier than creamy sauces and gravies. As a rule of thumb, red is usually better than white or yellow. Get all sauces, gravies and creams on the side so you can add to taste.

Dining Disasters

Restaurant dining can be especially tricky for tracking calorie intake. With the appetizer rolls, butter, cocktails, nuts, chips, and salsa, the "meal before the meal" can add an additional 700 calories to your total, sabotaging any effort for healthy dining.

Consider that a light beer carries about 100 calories, and at more than 100 calories an ounce, a few handfuls of nuts can add 500 to 600 more. You'll do better to skip the pre-meal snacking and ask your server about the size of the portions.

FOOD FOR THOUGHT: Entrée to win! Shake up the usual order of things in a restaurant by ordering your entrée before drinks or appetizers. This will take the edge off your appetite so that you'll order more modestly. Count on saving at least 400 calories per night out. Bottom line: If you "irritate the waiter" just once a week, that adds up to losing 6 pounds a year!

Customer's Always Right

Here are some questions I suggest that will help you eat healthier when you're eating at your favorite restaurant:

"Is this dish fried?"

"Can you make this dish without frying?"

"What is the sauce made with?"

"Can you prepare this without the cheese/sauce?"

"How large is the serving?"

"How many ounces is the beef, chicken, fish?"

"Can you make this dish without soy sauce or MSG?"

FOOD FOR THOUGHT: Don't hesitate to ask questions or make special requests because you are embarrassed. Remember, restaurants want you to be satisfied because your business is important to them -- so don't be afraid to ask.

No Time to Dine

Quick meals when you're on the go...

1. Peanut butter sandwich on whole wheat bread with a glass of milk and an apple.

2. Smallest fast food burger –with ketchup and mustard and a diet drink. Then when you get home –have an apple or baby carrots.

3. Precooked chicken strips and micro waved broccoli topped with a little cheese.

4. A healthy frozen entrée with a salad and glass of milk.

5.   Scrambled eggs with a vegetable of your choice and add whole wheat toast.

6.   Frozen vegetables micro waved –topped with Parmesan cheese and 2 Tablespoons of chopped nuts.

7.   Pre-bagged salad topped with canned tuna, with a little cheese, tomatoes and matchstick carrots.

8.   Sliced turkey from the deli on whole wheat bread with cheese, tomatoes and some mustard.

Keen Cuisines

We've all heard the saying "When in Rome, do as the Romans." Take heed of this and follow what the Italians have been eating for centuries. The **Mediterranean diet** styles itself with the eating habits of Southern Europeans including Greece. The "diet" consists of a high intake of fish, whole grains, fruits, nuts, vegetables and Olive oil. I'd advocate this type of plan everyday. Engage yourself into the healthy lifestyle of the ancient Greeks and Romans.

I'm going to give you some tips that you'll be able to use when you eat at your most popular eating establishments.

CHINESE

You can eat plenty of vegetables at any Chinese cuisine, but many of the dishes are high in greasy fat.

The Good:

2 cups Chicken / Steamed Vegetables with rice	490 cal	12 fat grams
2 cups Chicken Chop Suey with rice	600 cal	20 fat grams
1 cup Egg Drop soup	93 cal	5 fat grams
2 cups Stir-fried Broccoli and Carrots with rice	610 cal	28 fat grams

Not So Good:

2 cups Sweet and Sour Pork with rice	1529 cal 71 fat grams
8 ounces Spare Ribs	645 cal 43 fat grams
2 cups Kung Pao Chicken with rice	1210 cal 54 fat grams
2 cups Pork Fried Rice	710 cal 34 fat grams

ITALIAN

Go easy on all the extra cheese and fried foods. These extra goodies add up quickly and can spoil a usually healthy menu.

The Good:

1 cup Minestrone Soup	206 cal 5 fat grams
6 ounces Veal cutlet with peppers in sauce	488 cal 21 fat grams
2 cups Pasta Primavera	425 cal 20 fat grams
2 cups Pasta Fagioli (my favorite –pasta and beans)	300 cal 8 fat grams

Not So Good:

3 cups Fried Calamari w/tomato sauce	1077 cal 53 fat grams
2 cups Spinach and Cheese Tortellini	1260 cal 46 fat grams
2 cups Pasta in Pesto sauce	990 cal 56 fat grams
6 inch X 3 inch Meat Lasagna	625 cal 37 fat grams

MEXICAN

Normally very healthy dose of beans, rice and corn. It's when we add the fried tortillas and globs of cheese it gets unhealthy.

The Good:

1 cup Black Bean Soup	180 cal	5 fat grams
1 Chicken Fajita w/2 tbsp Salsa and 2 tbsp Guacamole	470 cal	26 fat grams
1 cup Yellow Rice and Black Beans	315 cal	1 fat gram
¼ cup Salsa	30 cal	2 fat grams

Not So Good:

1 Chicken Tostada w beans, Cheese, Sour Cream, Avocado	935 cal	55 fat grams
1 Taco Salad; Chicken, Rice, Lettuce, Rice, Beans, Tomatoes, Salsa, Guacamole in a Tortilla Shell	585 cal	48 fat grams
1 Cheese Quesadilla w/ Sour Cream, Salsa and Guacamole	900 cal	59 fat grams
10 large chips Nachos w/Beans and Cheese	800 cal	50 fat grams

ALL AMERICAN

We tend to deep fry our appetizers and add extra cheese toppings to many dishes. It still comes down to lowering the portion sizes when eating at an All-American fare.

The Good:

1 cup Chili Con Carne	300 cal	5 fat grams
4 ounces Grilled Fish w/ 1 tbsp Butter	196 cal	9 fat grams
3 ounces Barbecued Pork Chop w/2 tbsp Barbecue Sauce	202 cal	12 fat grams
3 ounces Grilled Chicken Breast w /one cup Vegetables	135 cal	4 fat grams

Not So Good:

3 Barbecued Ribs	1680 cal	144 fat grams
1 Cheeseburger w/Mushrooms	990 cal	57 fat grams
2 Jalapeno Poppers	660 cal	36 fat grams
6 Buffalo wings w ¼ cup Blue Cheese Dressing	1078 cal	68 fat grams

STEAK RESTAURANTS

You could ingest more fat in one sitting faster than you can say, "round em up –move em out." High quantities of fried, fattening foods and super size me portions usually characterize these places. However, I'll show you how to "chow down" without sabotaging your healthy habits.

The Good:

4 ounces Filet Mignon	192 cal	10 fat grams
6 Shrimp Cocktail w 2 tbsp Cocktail Sauce	158 cal	2 fat grams
4 ounces Broiled Salmon	171 cal	11 fat grams
1-¼ pounds Lobster in the Shell w/1 tbsp melted butter	325 cal	13 fat grams

Not So Good:

1 cup Creamed Spinach	290 cal	26 fat grams
16 ounces Porterhouse Steak	1300 cal	104 fat grams
1 cup Au gratin Potatoes	400 cal	22 fat grams
16 ounces Prime Rib	1170 cal	88 fat grams

SEAFOOD RESTAURANTS

If you can stay away from the deep fried, batter-dipped fish, you should be able to make very healthy, low-fat choices.

The Good:

5 large Peel and Eat Shrimp	114 cal	< 1 fat gram
4 ounces Grilled Swordfish	180 cal	10 fat grams
6 medium Oysters on the half Shell	120 cal	2 fat grams
4 ounces Red Snapper	144 cal	3 fat grams

Not So Good:

10 ounces Scallops with Fettuccine in Cream Sauce	1000 cal 61 fat grams
2 cups Fried Clams	900 cal 52 fat grams
6 Shrimp Scampi	932 cal 67 fat grams
4 ounces Fish and Chips	575 cal 27 fat grams

Life in the FAST LANE

You may have heard this in an earlier chapter …. "when I eat at fast food places ---I'm eating a lot of salads –how come I'm not losing weight!" Well, it's not in the lettuce or surrounding vegetables ---it's the high fat laden dressing that reverses your health gains of a salad. Let's take a look at some fast food salads.

Salads	Calories	Calories w/1 pkg dressing
MCDONALD'S		
Grilled Chicken Bacon Ranch Salad	270	560
Grilled Chicken California Cobb	280	400
Grilled Chicken Caesar	210	400
WENDY'S		
Chicken BLT Salad	310	590
Mandarin Chicken Salad	150	400
Southwest Chicken Caesar	260	480

As you can see, the salad dressing holds many calories. It's important NOT to douse your salads with dressing that has extra calories and fat. Remember, dip your fork in the dressing first, and then spear your food with fork that already has a sufficient amount of dressing on it. You're only interest is to have the taste. Or choose a fat-free dressing that is much lower in calories. As always, still watch your portions!

Better FAST FOOD Choices

These examples help to show that you can make better choices at fast food restaurants. BEWARE, if you are too tempted to order a "poor" choice, even though your intentions were to order a "better" choice, once you walk into a fast food restaurant, then you are wise to stay out! Visits to fast food restaurants should be occasional as opposed to regular.

Poor Choice	Better Choice
McDonald's	
Big Mac Sandwich	Grilled McChicken Sandwich*
Super Size French Fries	Side Salad w/ Low Fat Balsamic Vinaigrette
32 oz. Super Size Coke	8oz. low fat milk
1580 calories	**565 calories**
63 grams fat 22.5 grams fat	

To lower the fat even more leave off the sauce and add BBQ sauce instead.

Burger King

Double Whopper	BK Veggie
Large Onion Ring	Side salad
Zesty Dipping Sauce	Light Italian Dressing
Chocolate Shake	8oz. 1% milk
2240 calories	**520 calories**
135 grams fat	**17.5 grams fat**

Taco Bell

Burrito Supreme	Bean Burrito
Taco Salad	Soft Chicken Taco
2 oz. Large Pepsi	Water
1540 calories	**560 calories**
60 grams fat	**16 grams fat**

Wendy's

Big Bacon Classic	Spring Mix Salad w/ fat free French dressing and Small Chili
Biggie French Fries	
20 oz. large frosty	8 oz. low fat milk
1560 calories	**580 calories**
62 grams fat	**21 grams fat**

Pizza Hut

2 slices Stuffed Crust-Super Supreme	2 slices Thin N Crispy-Veggie Lovers
4 mild wings	1 piece garlic bread
1.5 oz. blue cheese dipping sauce	
Large Pepsi	Water
1610 calories	**530 calories**
78 grams fat	25 grams fat

If you like a certain type of fast food, like a double-decker hamburger, fried chicken, or a meat topped slice of pizza, than I would advise to balance the rest of the meal with a lower fat choice like a salad or a yogurt fruit parfait. Losing weight and living lean is all about total calories. Eat Smart!

Not sure how your favorite fast food menus fare? Most fast food restaurants have web sites that contain nutritional information on their foods. Check them out before you head off to the drive-thru!

Calorie and Fat

	Not So Good	Good	Savings
Burger King	Original Whopper 700 calories 39 fat grams	Hamburger 310 calories 12 fat grams	390 calories 27 fat grams
McDonald's	Big Mac 560 calories 30 fat grams	Hamburger 260 calories 9 fat grams	300 calories 21 fat grams
Wendy's	Big Bacon Classic 580 calories 29 fat grams	Jr. Hamburger 280 calories 9 fat grams	300 calories 20 fat grams

Good choices at fast food restaurants............

Baked Potatoes

Chicken sandwich –grilled

Chili –bowl

French Fries –small

Hamburgers –single

Milkshake –lowfat, small

Pizza –2 slices of 10" tossed crust (w/ vegetables)

Roast beef sandwich

Vegetable or grilled chicken salad -½ packet of dressing

Turkey sandwich

Yogurt –frozen with fruit topping

Wrap –turkey or chicken

Watch the toppings! That is what can get you into trouble. Try leaving off cheese, mayo and other high fat sandwich toppers.

COMMENDABLE CONDIMENTS: Be picky here. These little dressings can make or break your caloric count for the day. These are my favorites, because I know they're very low in fat and some are low in calories.

Ketchup 2 tbsp = 30 cal

Mustard   2 tbsp = 32 cal

Horseradish   1 tbsp =6 cal

Whipped Butter 1 tbsp = 70 cal

Light margarine 1 tbsp = 20 cal

Barbeque Sauce 2 tbsp = 40 cal

Steak Sauce 1 tbsp = 15 cal

Salsa   2 tbsp = 15 cal

Balsamic vinegar   1 tbsp = 2 cal

There's no such thing as "BAD" foods ----the food can either be Healthy or not as Healthy. So, Choose well.

FOOD FOR THOUGHT : Say no to food pushers! Take a positive approach. Sample the offered food, but tell your host, "This is great. I'd love to have more, but I'm very satisfied and can't take another bite." Be positive, yet firm.

Special Occasions

Most parties are surrounded by food. This doesn't mean you're going to sabotage your lean lifestyle. You just have to be prepared.

It's very important to realize that you can function at any party or holiday with a little bit of preplanning. Before any Holiday sneaks up on you, create a plan on how you're going to incorporate fitness and healthy nutrition into your daily routine.

I have always found that if I know I have a big day of eating ahead of me—Thanksgiving comes to mind, I make sure that I eat regularly all day long. If the party is in the afternoon-don't forget to eat breakfast. Don't show up starving!

There's probably going to be finger foods, sweets and fattening entrees at your party. Here are a few tricks to help you stay true to your health goals while enjoying the festivities.

- Make you're first helping small-your host will always expect you to have two servings. This will help with your portion control
- Don't stand next to the food table
- Wear tighter fitting outfits – that will give you no room for expansion
- Give leftover food away to neighbors, family or take it to work as a leftover
- If you're at a buffet table- decide on three or four favorites and only make one high in calories
- Bring a healthy dish with you so that you know there will be something safe to eat. I'll bet there will be other people there that will be just as happy that you did
- Conversation is **calorie free**. Talk with your friends and family members
- You're there for the celebration …….NOT THE FOOD
- Socialize away from the display of food
- Don't arrive at parties ravenous. Eat or drink before you meet. Have a glass of water or a serving of fruit or vegetable
- Select a bite size sampling of several of the deserts or appetizers-not one huge piece

- Don't waste all your calories on alcohol
- When in doubt, always give yourself a little "wiggle" room with your calories. If I know that I'm going out to eat dinner with friends at a special restaurant, I won't eat as many calories during the day, but I still eat!
- Make a plan. If you do what you always do –you'll get what you always get. There has to be some alteration to get a healthy response
- When you feel thirsty, add ice to your drink, so you won't drink as much
- Learn the art of saying "no thanks"
- Don't squander calories. If you don't like Egg Nog---don't drink it. That goes for anything else
- If you like Aunt Rita's coconut Crème pie –eat it. But, skip the mashed potatoes and rolls

FOOD FOR THOUGHT: The average person gains between 5-7 pounds from Thanksgiving to New Years. Think about the reason. You're more likely to celebrate with family and friends at parties, and we find it easy to diminish our exercise plan for those 49 days leading up to New Years. Go for a walk in the mall during the holiday season. This is one time where you don't want to be "above " average.

Smart shopping

While food shopping, think **SMALL**: packages of single-serving-size cereals, crackers, cheeses, yogurts and snacks will help you with portion control.

Learn to buy on the outside of the grocery store where you find the vegetables, fruits and lean meats and dairy products. Also learn to travel down the aisles that have beans, legumes, and whole grain breads and cereals.

Chapter 6
HEALTHY STATE OF MIND-
Deflecting All Obstacles

OBSTACLE # 1-Lack of a Goal

There are many obstacles that can block you from success. You may have run into the lack of a **goal**. What do you really want? I need you to be specific here. Don't just say I want to lose weight and firm up a little. That's too general. How about " I want to drop 3 pant sizes." Or "I want to be able to walk up to 15 minutes without breathing hard." I want to be able to participate in a line dance by the end of the year." Be specific.

Only you really know what you want out of life. It's up to you to set your goals. It was Napoleon Hill who said, "What the mind can conceive and believe, the mind can **achieve** with a positive mental attitude." I want you to become enthusiastic towards your goal. Your enthusiasm should make reaching that goal a burning **desire**. That's where I need your thought patterns to be: burning desire to succeed.

I want to share a story with you about a young woman who had a burning desire to live a normal life, instead of one that was filled with pain, frustration and all of the other negative associations for someone who is over-fat. Her name is Donna Rosen. When I first met her she was 317 pounds and she told me that her desire was to live a normal life and that she would do **anything** to get there. Her other desire was to dance with Patrick Swayze. Get down Donna. Just like you, Donna had the same ingredients to change her way of thinking. The same ingredients I've given you. After 25 years of diets that had failed her, Donna now is a normal 158 pounds and loving life, all because Donna had that burning desire to succeed.

When she slipped up along the way, she realized that it was just one day and tomorrow was another day that she could commit to being healthy. Donna's not a model-- she's just like you and me — a normal person who's taking simple, necessary steps to reprogram her lifestyle. It works!

Remember, success is a journey, not a destination.

I need you to focus on the process, not the end result. Donna took the weight off one pound at a time. If she had tried losing 150 pounds all at once, then it would have been overwhelming. Donna broke her goal down into small attainable goals. By the way, Donna is still living this journey and will not be satisfied until she hits her goal weight of 135. Donna is adamant about that number! She wanted to fit into the same dress she did when she got married. I have all the confidence that she'll do it because she has a **burning desire** and she's not afraid of making a few mistakes along the way. Donna confronted her fears of failure and said, "I'm never heading back to where I was."

You can figure if you've had a slight gain of pounds, it's OK. Just get back on the right track again and follow my 15 Ways…one way at a time. You'll lose body fat and increase muscle tissue, which will guarantee you long-term success and permanent weight management. I think a common notion is that some of the successful people you read about, like Donna, who lost 158 pounds, or Mary Ella who lost 50 pounds, or Jodi who lost 40 pounds are "gifted" people or they're doing something different than you or I. The truth is, people who have gone through the program with specific goals in mind, and a burning desire to succeed, make these success stories. So, set realistic goals and then enjoy the process. Hitting the target is fabulous…but don't forget to enjoy the journey as well.

OBSTACLE # 2 Floundering Fitness

Dreadful, Hassle, Distressful, Punishment. Is this a penitentiary or do these words describe your attitude towards exercise?

You're probably sitting there saying to yourself, "you've got me convinced I need to do some exercise - I think." You realize all the benefits of starting a plan; but you still have a little doubt. If I had a crystal ball that viewed all the successful people who ever lost weight and kept it off, then the one proven element that keeps resurfacing would be physical activity.

Oh, I know you're very busy, I understand your dilemma- I've been there. I spent the first 5 years of my daughter's life as Mr. Mom. I ran my business out of my home. I can fully understand that you have to be your child's teacher, cook, playmate, guidance counselor and it doesn't leave a lot of time to "get physical."

However, once you do squeeze fitness into your jam-packed schedule, your life will begin to open up, because you'll become more efficient – mentally as well as physically at everything you do. Can you think of a better way to add more hours to your day than that?

It seems the more hours we spend working HARD – the SOFTER we become. You have a choice, and now you will make the time – even if it's a little bit here and a little bit there. Remember, the studies showed that exercise is accumulative – it all adds up.

If you're used to being inactive, then I know how tough it must seem to make this commitment to yourself. You'll have to change your outlook, as well as your behavior. I want you to understand that fitness shouldn't be this unrealistic regimen, inflexible, or overly complicated – it should be FUN! Yes FUN – this isn't penance. Your body was meant to move – think back when you were younger. You were constantly moving and not worrying about your body.

To make weight loss work with your busy lifestyle – you're not only going to have to learn to use your body, but you're going to have to learn to use your imagination. The greatest thing you should realize, when you're just starting to become active is that the person who benefits the

most is the person who has been doing it the **least.** You're going to feel wonderful.

You've done a lot of thinking about becoming a vibrant, healthy, energetic person: You know it's the right thing to do for your health, especially when your Doctor keeps harping at you to start. You know it's going to improve your looks- just by doing a little. NOW is the time to act.

Listed below are different ways to change your daily routine to become more active. Choose two changes that you're ready to commit in each category. Remember, choose only the ones in which you can truly have an opportunity to do.

To become more active at home

____ I will use the phone furthest from where I am
____ I will "lose" the TV remote
____ I will do one extra cleaning or gardening every week
____ I will do housework with a little more "elbow grease"
____ I will take a short walk at least once a day
     -to the mailbox, or to visit friends
____ I have my own idea of how to become more active
     I will _____

To become more active at work

____ I will walk to the furthest bathroom – at a brisk pace!
____ I will walk to speak to co-workers rather than call on the phone
____ I will use part of my lunch hour to get some exercise
____ I will stand when I use the phone
____ I will take active coffee breaks -----walking instead of sitting
____ I have my own idea of how to become more active
     I will _____

To become more active during free time

____ I will carry the groceries to the car myself
____ When I wait for an appointment, I will walk around rather than sit
____ I will run my own errands rather than letting others do them for me

___ I will walk or ride a bike to nearby errands
___ I will plan active family outing instead of passive ones
___ I will invite friends to do active things like dancing or a nature hike
___ I have my own idea of how to be more active
     I will _____

I want you to succeed more than anything. I know that at some point, even your best plans seem to be side-railed. We must handle these roadblocks even before they come up. Look over the examples below and figure out what you would do about these roadblocks.

Stumble # 1: You have decided that you're going to start walking a few blocks after dinner. However, tonight, it's really cold out there.
What do you think? What do you say to yourself?

_____

_____

_____

_____

_____

_____

Stumble # 2: You've decided to get more activity by parking further away from the mall entrance (isn't that annoying when people drive around for minutes just to find a closer space?)

Your partner says, "Don't park so far away. I don't feel like walking this far." What do you do? What do you say?

_____

_____

_____

_____

_____

_____

Stumble # 3: You've made up your mind that you're going to start taking the stairs at work. A co-worker says to you: "Why take the stairs, what are you a health nut?" What do you do? What do you say?

_____

_____

_____

_____

Stumble # 4: You decided that yard work and gardening will provide you with more activity. However, today is your day and your back feels a little achy. What do you think? What can you say to yourself?

_____

_____

_____

_____

OBSTACLE # 3 –Lack of Motivation

Another important part of your journey is rewarding yourself along the way. Obstacle # 3 can hinder your progress by the lack of motivation or lack of <u>rewards</u>. You need to create, nurture and update a well-planned motivational system. It's easy to stay focused when you control your levels of motivation with the help of a reward system. Why do you or don't you exercise? Why do you or don't you eat healthy? Why do you spend hours on the phone? Our behaviors don't lie. Everything we do serves a purpose and that purpose usually makes us feel good.

This is important: Reward yourself every step of the way as soon as possible and keep rewarding yourself until the change becomes a habit. There is no need to wait until you reach your goal before you reap the benefits of weight loss.

For example, Jayne Niemela has lost 25 pounds. She buys herself a new CD every time she takes off 5 pounds. A friend of mine, Rick Malizia, a loser of 30 pounds, treats himself to a game of golf when he stays on his nutrition plan for a week. Think about the treats you can give yourself for accomplishing your mini-goals. Your rewards may be free or involve your spouse or a friend. The rewards may take less than a minute. They could be mental or spiritual rather than physical. Rewards have no boundaries.

A word of caution - don't use food as a reward. For instance, I knew a young woman in Florida who used to workout with me and at the end of each week she would go to McDonalds and have a small bag of fries and a milkshake. That was her way of patting herself on the back for a hard week's worth of training. She was sabotaging her efforts to reach her goals! Every change you make on your journey, from eating portion-controlled foods to popping in your exercise dvd's every week is an accomplishment.

It's very important for you to keep the process of change marching forward in a positive direction by rewarding yourself. Since it may take awhile for you to reach your ultimate body- giving yourself rewards along the way will boost your motivation to stay with your new habits. Begin by giving yourself short-term rewards after you accomplish short-term goals, such as, walking 25 minutes today. Plan for long-term rewards after accomplishing **monthly** goals like losing 2 inches in your hips.

<u>**TAKE CHARGE NOW.**</u> Your outlook and attitude towards your self will determine how successful my plan will work for you.

I hope you can answer <u>**YES**</u> to most of these statements:

- I do my exercises –even when I don't feel like getting active
- I know I can keep this lifestyle up if I WANT TO
- I am the only one who can decide be active or be a couch potato
- I make commitments to eat healthy on a daily basis and then I fulfill them
- I schedule exercise on a regular basis
- I am proud of the way I am approaching my healthy lifestyle
- I don't let other issues affect my healthy lifestyle
- I don't make excuses for not being active
- I like when other people admire my new lifestyle

OBSTACLE # 4 Impatience
(expecting too much too soon)

Another obstacle is impatience - wanting the pounds to drop off too quickly. If you equate success with fast weight loss, then you may fail on this plan. I don't believe in giving you something I know doesn't work. This is not a "hey, give us a week and we'll take off 15 pounds" program. Those programs are dangerous! In the beginning of my plan, you will lose more weight in the first few weeks, but then it will taper off as I teach you the strategies to keep it off permanently.

A few years ago, I ran into a distant cousin of mine, who I hadn't seen in 20 years. I knew her as an overweight, young woman who probably needed to lose 100 pounds. Well, let me tell you when I saw her I hardly recognized her. She looked awful! She was 47 but looked 67. She lost over 80 pounds; but she did it by starving herself. I mean her face looked gaunt and sunk in. She did not look healthy. When you lose weight by not eating, you lose muscle and not much fat. As I told you before, the scale can be very deceptive.

As you put on muscle tissue you may even gain some weight. However, the weight you gain will not be coming from fat. You may think this is awful because your goal was to lose weight-not gain it. Remember, muscle is great, because it burns calories faster than fat. After a short period of time, your metabolism will increase as you replace fat with muscle. But it does take a little time for this to happen. So, take my advice – and don't beat yourself up over the scale – just remember – MORE MUSCLE = LESS FAT!!

Instead, maybe set a goal of moving your belt over one notch or being able to zip up that beautiful summer dress or that favorite old pair of jeans you haven't been able to get into. Be patient with me, and have confidence in me. Do it my way... the sensible, realistic way, and I promise that you'll look great, feel energetic and want to attack life with vim and vigor. Life is short. I don't need you to go through life at 70 percent. I need you to commit 100% of yourself towards success.

Let me give you another example of how quick weight loss can sabotage your long-term goals. Let's say you needed to lose 10 quick pounds in one week for your 20th high school reunion -So, you starved yourself and knew the weight would definitely come back-but you didn't care. Instead, you wanted to look great and show your high school boyfriend what he missed out on all these years. This instant gratification process will continue throughout your life if you don't put a stop to this negative thinking. It's not right to want such fast results in return for so very little effort.

An all-or-nothing attitude is why so many people have so little success; we choose structured programs because they relieve us from making choices for ourselves. A properly designed program makes sense, but expecting to stick to a structured eating and exercise plan for an extended period of time without ever deviating makes no sense at all. In fact, this is so unrealistic, it's set-up for failure from the start. If you begin to change your habits with the assumption that any deviation from your plan will ruin it, then you might as well not even start. Life is full of unplanned obstacles, distractions, and temptations. Your best approach is to prepare for them by keeping an open mind and maintaining a positive attitude.

It was **Epiclesis** who said, "Nothing comes into existence all at once, not even the grape, or the fig. If you say to me now, 'I want a fig,' I shall answer, 'that requires time.' Let the tree blossom first, then put forth its fruit and finally let the fruit ripen."

Your journey will have one struggle after another, but it will happen for you. Sometimes it may take a little gratification in sight until you finally reach your goal and enjoy your rewards. To rise above, you must realize that the fruits of success ripen slowly, and often after repeated errors.

Let me share with you my personal story on waiting my turn. After leaving a successful personal training business in Florida, which I nurtured for five years, I moved back to my hometown in Ohio. I left a job, a beautiful home, and relocated. I started from scratch. That's a lot of stress at one time in anyone's life.

I will tell you that I vowed to myself that I would be a success and that my new venture would bring me to a new personal career level. I had some success with my sales of my videos on Home Shopping Network and Direct Response TV. Still, after three years and plenty of managerial mistakes, my business was not where I wanted it. But, I never stopped believing in myself and took each business experience and chalked it up as a learning experience and when one door opened there were five that shut.

And just like you're going to do, I hung in there and tried harder. I had a burning desire. I told myself to keep going – just move forward. I persevered and through all my learning experiences and positioning myself, I found a wonderful marketing company who took my concepts and ideas and made them come to fruition. You can learn from my example of hitting a few snags along the way-just keep going. Winners never quit and quitters never win. Nobody stops you – but you! So be patient…keep at it…and enjoy the ride.

Lose weight –not patience!

OBSTACLE # 5   A Stumble is Not a Tumble

Let's say you were on your GET LEAN IN 15 eating plan for two weeks and then you "slipped" and had a few unhealthy meals. You're feeling terrible. You know what I say? **Who cares** if you slip once in awhile! You're human! Let's look at this way you're still way ahead of the game. Two weeks of eating, that's roughly 70 chances (snacks included) to eat and you goofed 10 times, that's 60 to 10 –you WIN! You're a success! Give yourself some credit, pat yourself on the back, and get back on the plan.

Rather than expecting perfection and viewing lapses as total catastrophes, recognize setbacks as valuable opportunities to learn and to identify problems and develop strategies for the future. This "all or nothing" attitude is probably the very reason why most people fail to keep weight off. Your GET LEAN IN 15 meal plan was designed to teach you how to make healthy choices. I *never* expect you to stick to the plan 100% of the time. It's meant to work *with* you so it doesn't disrupt your lifestyle.

I don't want you to think that if you deviate from your menus that you blew it and failed, and ruined your journey. It's OK. A slip is not a fall. There are a lot of things that will come up. For example, a business luncheon with the boss; Suzie's birthday; a vacation in Florida; you're sick; the kids need to eat and it's 5:30; and you head to a fast food place. It's OK! These occurrences are always going to pop up.

Prepare for them mentally by saying to yourself that its 'just one day.' Then accept it and move on. Tomorrow will be a victory day. Don't let one day ruin your journey, get right back on the plan as soon as possible, and keep the progress of change moving forward.

If you find yourself diving into the Godiva chocolate box, enjoy them. Savor the taste. Hey, eat a couple for me. I want you to feel good that you weren't out of control. You didn't deprive yourself and you're back on track. I never want you to feel that I'm depriving you of the foods you enjoy…remember, it's how much you eat that's the problem. Calories count!

If you deprive yourself, then a natural response will be "Hey Jaime, I'll show you, you health nut, take your chicken breast sandwich and shove it. I'm going with the Philly cheese-steak sandwich with extra cheese. " That's rebellious and it's not going to help you with long-term results. I want you to take that "all or nothing" approach and replace it with a calm, non-incriminating way of eating and exercising.

Take a look at some of the successful people that you know. Do you think that they've slipped a few times? Sure they did! Do you think the next "hot" new actor or actress makes it overnight? You may think they do because of a one hit movie, but believe me, nine times out of ten, they never tell you how many times they failed and had to wait on tables for a living.

If you think you blew it, then keep in mind, that it's not a setback – just a part of the process. It can be viewed as a signal for you to be especially kind and loving towards yourself, as if you were consoling a close friend or a family member. Offer yourself the same support, encouragement or acceptance.

For example, you go to the store and you're buying your week's worth of groceries from your list, and all of a sudden the Sara Lee chocolate cake starts calling your name. So, you buy it and eat a couple slices and you feel guilty. Specifically, you feel, "Oh my gosh, I'm terrible. I'm a failure. I really blew it. I can't stick with anything!" Your good advice to yourself would be, "OK, so I ate a couple pieces of cake. It's over. I can succeed if I get back on my program right now!!"

OBSTACLE # 6   Negative Nay Sayer

Okay, obstacle # 6 is a big one...negative self-talk. Beating yourself up with that powerful little voice in your head. Every once in awhile we use self-defeating chatter in our mind. You say to yourself, "I'm too fat" or "I'm not good enough."

Negative self-talk can develop into an unhealthy pattern. Here's what you can do about it, you can start by developing positive mind chatter by taking the negative statement, "I'm too fat," and turning it into, "I'm the perfect weight for me at this time." It may sound simplistic, even absurd. Let's analyze this. First, notice that I didn't say, "I'm the perfect weight." I said, "I'm the perfect weight **for me** at this time." It suggests that I might get to another perfect weight later on.

When you find that you're feeling badly about yourself, ask yourself "what beliefs am I acting on?" What has my self-talk been that has produced such feelings? What negative thought pattern have I slipped into?

SAY the RIGHT things to yourself.
- Make a firm decision to change
- Become aware of the irrational or negative thought ---identify it
- Take time to ponder that negative thought

   YOU NEVER FAIL --UNLESS YOU STOP TRYING!!

When you find yourself thinking negative thoughts about yourself, just remember the visual cue of a stop sign! Immediately, replace the negative with a positive. I've always heard that if you don't have something nice to say, then don't say anything at all. This rule should apply to the most important person in the world: YOU!

Being successful starts in your mind. It was Frank Outlaw who said,
- **Watch your thoughts, they become words.**
- **Watch your words, they become actions.**
- **Watch your actions, they become your habits.**
- **Watch your habits, they become your character.**
- **Watch your character, it becomes your destiny.**

Think about it. I want to hear you telling yourself, "I'm tired of beating myself up, and I know that if I follow the **FIT15 plan**, then I believe I'm capable of doing it. I'm going to march forward and do my best…and have a daily victory every day! If I slip, then it's no big deal. I'll just keep persevering. I'm not going to let my fears get the best of me. I'm in this game for the long run. This time I will succeed." I want you to think of this process like an old record. You can keep playing the same broken record of the past, reliving past problems, pitying yourself for past mistakes; all of which, fuel negative self-feelings and failure. Or, you can choose to put on a new record, one that makes you feel good about you.

The new record has a framework for success and that winning feeling, which will help you do better everyday and get you one step closer to your goal. Bottom line- if you don't like the music, and then change the tune!!

OBSTACLE # 7 Fear

Fear of failure and even fear of success. Very often we procrastinate because we believe we may fail at our goal. A perfect example of this is when we walk into an aerobic class and take a look around and see all these energetic people bouncing around in their spandex outfits, having fun and keeping perfect count with the instructor. So what do we do?

We get intimidated, nervous and feel there is no way we're going to embarrass ourselves and feel inadequate.

The fear of failure can hold us back in our quest for total success. I say jump in with both feet and go for it. You'd be surprised to know that most people wouldn't even notice or even care if you were in the room, because they're too busy worrying about themselves. If you feel gyms are intimidating and frightening for you, then purchase exercise dvd's and work out in the privacy and convenience of your own home. Problem solved! Personal growth requires that you take some risks. They say progress involves risks -you can't steal second base with your foot on first.

Now, let's talk about a different fear -**the fear of success.** You're probably thinking that's ridiculous, how could I undermine my own progress of something that I want so badly? Remember this, no one likes to find their self in such an unfamiliar territory. You could fear that your new body will bring on something so vague as a simple compliment. You have to turn your emotional dial and switch to pleasure and winning- instead of possibly spending a lifetime of criticisms and insults. That was your old way of thinking. As you stop using your old patterns you may feel emptiness-almost like you lost a friend.

You may feel a little anxiety about your new look. You may wonder what life is like as a person at your goal weight. Will you feel like a different person? Will there be social demands? You may say, " I want to change -it's just too scary." You may need to take steps to find out what's scaring you. Being honest with yourself is the best way to overcome fear. As you face your own fears, they're less likely to have a hold on you. This kind of thinking prevents you from taking a chance and being fit.

Your new way of thinking has to say, "it's time for me to do it now- not tomorrow -now." Failure can be like a roadmap, clearly marking what avenues you want to avoid. Watch out for those detours. They'll become guidelines or instruction about where NOT to go next time.

When you reach your goal, there is still another fear of success that can rear its ugly head. Having gone through the journey to being fit, you may now worry that you won't be able to KEEP the weight off. You may live in fear that you can't match the fit body that you have discovered. Rest assured, that I have given you all the tools in my plan for lifetime weight management. Keep following the principles, and you will permanently keep the weight from returning.

I coined a term while I was in college called the "rise above theory." The concept is very simple -try to be "complete" in body, soul and mind, and you will achieve your goals and avoid the fear of failure.

I must share with you a personal story showing you how I put this into practice. I noticed most of the college kids around me were drinking and staying out late-typical college antics. Putting the theory of positive mental attitude to work, I realized that if I put in the time and effort, I could "rise above" the norm of what a college kid was supposed to accomplish. So, I would get up at 4:30 every morning, go to the gym, eat breakfast, go to classes and then go to a T.V. station and work as an intern during the evening. My life was filled with obstacles-perhaps just like yours; however, my mindset was one that I couldn't fail. I knew discipline, dedication and determination would pay off and it did. Today, I have helped millions of people all over the country get motivated to be fit. I learned that getting through your obstacles might take a little sacrifice; however, you will always WIN in the long run.

To "rise above" means to ignore that fear of failure or success. Move ahead. Stay with your new habits. You will become comfortable with your new body. If you're having trouble keeping the weight off, then remind yourself how hard you worked and the length of time that you were able to maintain your new body. Then get right back to your new habits. My plan allows you leeway for trial and error patterns, because you know you can survive setbacks and you will take risks and try new things. I need you to just keep trying and trying – your hours of work and eating smart will continue to bring you success.

OBSTACLE # 8 Dependency

One reason you may not be reaching your full potential is an obstacle... called dependency. Get in shape for yourself only- don't do it for anyone else. Your old ways of thinking would have you believing this negative self-image of yourself turning to other people or other things because of feeling of inadequacy.

What dependency does is deprive you of your own freedom to choose your own course of action leading towards personal growth and fulfillment. I was training a young woman in Los Angeles, and her exercise sessions were going great. However, when I left for a vacation, she couldn't handle the situation of me not being there for her. So she ate profusely and didn't do her workouts. She was holding herself back because she was co-dependent on our training sessions. She felt she couldn't do it by herself. I confronted her with this and she denied it. I had to drop her as a client… for her own good. I never saw her in the gym again.

I don't want this to happen to you. Follow **Get Lean In 15** just for YOU. You want it badly. It's your body. You're the one that's going to benefit. Not your spouse, not your family members, not your friends – Do it for YOU.

Family members and friends will be in your life as you make this journey to health; however, sometimes these people along your path may NOT want you to succeed, possibly because of their own insecurities. It could be jealously or it could be concern over their own weight. They could sabotage your efforts by saying, "I want the old Suzie back. She was a lot more fun. She used to go out drinking all the time or have a large popcorn at the movies with extra butter." You're not alone when you feel these comments hurt, even though you may know that these people probably wish they could be as committed as you are. You may even want to apologize for your efforts.

Don't be fooled, there's no NEED to feel guilty or discouraged by your own health successes. You're doing great and no one has the right to undermine your goals. If someone does make you feel uncomfortable with their comments, you can ignore their remarks. You can give the person the benefit of the doubt and realize that they don't know how to express themselves or how to be supportive. You can stand up for YOU yourself. Turn those hurtful remarks into healthy reactions. You can control the situation.

If you're ever feeling a little down because you've reached a plateau with your weight or you've fallen off the plan or missed a goal…I want you to watch other people who have succeeded at losing weight and keeping it off. They are great role models for you. Listen to their stories. Listen to their struggles. You can probably relate to them and learn from them.

This journey of being fit involves learning about your thoughts, feelings, and attitudes about food and fitness in a very special way. You will learn NEW WAYS to reshape old habits around eating and activity.

Imagine trying to lose weight while your husband, wife, family or friends are constantly trying to get you to eat fattening things. They may try to convince you, "It's okay to eat that -- it's your birthday, anniversary, the weekend or…. any excuse." Or perhaps they keep telling you, "You're fine just the way you are, you don't need to lose weight." Your so-called "support group" may not want to see you "suffer" through yet another diet. They may even be trying to sabotage your efforts because they are jealous or feel guilty of your new lifestyle choices.

On the other hand, study after study has shown how solid family and social networks can positively influence your health. It's not a leap of faith to infer that strong support from family and friends brings "an increase in self-confidence" by validating the individual's choice to lose weight, a reduction in overall stress, and increased attention to achieving the overall goal of good health.

OBSTACLE # 9 Lack of Time

One reason why people may fail to reach their goals is that sometimes we bite off a little more than we can chew. If you feel you have too many things to do, it may be because you really do have…. too many things to do. Are you the type that can't say "no" and so you end up doing the work of three people? Stand in the mirror and practice your "no" and say it gently but firmly when the need rises.

Trying to lose weight is stressful, so try to resolve other sources of stress in your life before you begin your weight loss attempt-this will give you your best chance for success. For instance, if you were planning on throwing a wedding party, now would not be the best time to concentrate on your weight loss program. Remember, there's a big difference between waiting for the appropriate time in your life and sheer procrastination.

It's wise to examine your motivation, your commitment and stress levels. By making sure that these factors are in order your weight loss program will be littered with less than ideal times and when the going gets tough, you'll have to really bear down on all your physical and mental resources at a moments notice. But, don't wait until life is perfect either, because, let's face it, you'll be waiting for a long time.

With GET LEAN IN 15, even if you're strapped for time, you still can do it. Think about how your really spend your time. On a piece of paper, I want you to divide your day into three parts.

1. Waking up through Lunch
2. End of Lunch to Dinner
3. End of Dinner until you go to sleep

How do you fill up these segments of your day? For instance, you may spend 30 minutes getting ready for work, 20 minutes eating breakfast, having your coffee and reading the paper. How many minutes do you spend talking on the phone? shopping? cooking? taking naps? watching TV? socializing? daydreaming?

My point is simple; from your time management list you can see patterns in your lifestyle on how your valuable time is spent. I know if you work at home or have a job outside the home that accounts for at least eight hours. You may sleep for another six-eight hours. Well then, you can use eight-ten hours of your day for yourself.

I created the workouts to fit into your schedule. You can't give the excuse for lack of time. I KNOW you have 15 minutes! There's days when I can't get a complete workout-but—I do something—and now you can too –you deserve that time for yourself.

Your life is divided into 24 separate 60-minute vignettes every day. How you choose to divide your "portions" will effect every part of who you are. When you're trying to control your weight, there are key issues that must be addressed to be successful. We all live within the same 24-hour time zone- me, you, your neighbor, and even the President of the United States.

We know that lean people lead lean lives. What makes these individuals succeed when others fail? It's how they choose to live their 'slices of life.' Life is about choices.

OBSTACLE # 10 The Plateau

We've all had them. Our body reaches these natural set points and doesn't want to budge –up or down. Don't get discouraged, this is a natural phase in the journey towards weight management. A former client of mine, Laurie Guerini, lost a total of 86 pounds using my system. During the last 20 pounds of her goal weight, Laurie became distraught that her weight was not moving down as quick. Her body seemed to be "holding" on to those last few stubborn pounds. In her mind, Laurie thought that she reached a "plateau." She began to lose the enthusiasm and started to slide in her pledge to her goal. Her desire to keep losing was equal to her desire to eat more food and not be as committed to exercise. Sound familiar?

This happens quite often. You've lost enough to be satisfied, but not quite enough to reach your goal weight. Even if you're at the beginning of your journey, you may be tempted to not be as healthy. You've lost a few pounds and your motivation to stick closely to your healthy menus slips a little –this is the time that you need to forget about all those past relapses and jump right back into the plan.

Breaking the Plateau:

1. Change your exercise routine. Start at the end of your exercise sequence instead of the beginning. Increase the repetitions or increase the resistance. Walk for an extra 15 minutes every day for a week. Your body needs to be challenged to progress, so make sure you're changing some part of your program every 4-6 weeks.

2. Focus on your healthy choices you make that day, that week. You're more likely to stick with the plan knowing that you have these "Daily Victories."

3. Give yourself new rewards that you haven't tried yet. That mini vacation looks good about now.

4. Be specific with your daily changes. Today, I'm going to eat four pieces of fruit. Tomorrow, I'm going to have broccoli for lunch and dinner.

5. Make sure you're eating enough food. I know this sounds crazy. But, to jump-start your metabolism again –you may need to eat more food. If your body doesn't have enough fuel to sustain your level of activity, you can actually stop losing weight. Don't starve yourself-you have to eat to lose!

6. Get off the scale. Concentrate on the way your new body feels. Pay close attention to the way your clothes are fitting.

7. Start writing down everything you're eating. Are there sneaky little calories that are coming in that you're not paying attention to?

8. USE THE LEAN PLATE to get back to proper portions.

9. Drink only water as your beverage for the next week and see if that makes a difference.

10. Stop exercising so much. When you increase your exercise intensity, your body responds by decreasing the amount of calories you burn during the rest of your day. If you reach exercise burnout, this is a great time to take a break for a few days, or try something gentle like yoga or a stretching routine. After you've rested, get back to exercise-but lighten up your original routine and increase your intensity only as necessary.

Almost everyone reaches a weight loss plateau at some point. As your body adapts to your workouts, it becomes more efficient at it and, therefore, doesn't expend as many calories doing it. You may find that after your initial weight loss, your progress will slow down and eventually stop.

SET POINT THEORY – each of us has an "internal regulator" much like a thermostat that fights to keep a certain weight.

If you eat <u>too many</u> calories –the SET POINT kicks up your metabolism to maintain body fat levels. This can make you overweight!

If you eat <u>too little</u> calories, the set point <u>slows down</u> your metabolism to conserve energy in an attempt to maintain your weight. This can make you overweight!

OBSTACLE # 11 Stress

In your life, there are factors that you can control-and factors that you can't. Try to keep issues in your life in proper perspective. Try not to get stressed out over things beyond your control. I always ask my wife-what's the worst possible thing that could happen in any given situation—and that usually puts the mini problem in a different framework and helps ease the stress.

Everyone has stress; it's how we handle the stress that is the issue. Maintaining a healthy lifestyle is stressful if you're trying to be perfect at it.

Nobody's perfect!

Perfectionism can be your worst enemy in trying to eat healthy every meal or trying to exercise daily. Perfectionism can turn the already large task of choosing healthier foods into the *overwhelming* task of finding the *perfect* food choice every single meal. This task becomes daunting. Nothing's good enough for you. Therefore, you may not even start it. Or, you may start a program, but when things start to go wrong -you eventually give up because it didn't meet your expectations. This can be a challenge. Though it's a process that may take a little time, shedding the burden of perfectionism can greatly decrease the level of stress you feel on a daily basis.

If you're struggling with perfectionism, you probably have tortured yourself by pointing out all of your mistakes or thinking that you don't want to start a weight management plan because you can't do it well enough. While this habit may be difficult to just stop, I need you to take some moments and think of all the good, positive things in your life. If you notice something about yourself that you don't like-take the time and find at least three other attributes that are good for you.

Perfectionists leave no margin for error. If you're too rigid in your goal setting or your meal planning, it's difficult when you hit a snag –which you will- by the way. Don't be so hard on yourself or judgmental. We all make mistakes. Remember, I discussed that you can still see excellent results even if you followed my eating plan 80 percent of the time. That's not perfect –but it works. This is precisely why my plan is real. You can still slip up and still succeed.

I knew a young fitness trainer in Florida who was a perfectionist regarding her workout schedule and eating habits. She was so obsessed about her routines that she would spend up to four hours in the gym daily either teaching or working herself out. She couldn't let go of the fact that she didn't have to train that hard to see results. She needed to have the perfect body –right now. Well guess what, that was a disaster waiting to happen…. and it did. She became so obsessed about her perfect body that she couldn't function in the real world. The gym fired her. Her clients left her and she literally fell apart and stopped going to the gym all together.

Think about how much happier, more productive, and less stressed you would be if you gave yourself a little break. I'm giving you permission to let go of the perfectionism-it leads to too much stress.

Dealing with stress can be as simple as taking a few minutes a day to take a mini vacation at your work desk or in your home. I have ALWAYS found that exercising is the perfect stress buster on several levels.

First, when you exercise, you release endorphins, that help soothe your mood. However, more importantly, no matter how much stress, or how bad my day is going, I know when I work out, that I'm doing something good for me. This alone, alleviates some of the stress that occurs over a problem. The problem might still be there –but you'll have better coping skills because of your attitude. Try it out next time you are faced with a confrontation.

Try to simplify your life immediately. Our lives are loaded with projects, goals, ideas, have-to commitments, concerns, and responsibilities.

Start by cutting out a few things that are not necessary. Give someone else the work to do or make a system for tasks that are sucking your energy stores dry.

When you think of something you "have to do," stop and ask yourself why you have to do it. You probably don't.

Choose habits that you WANT to do. There is no place for shoulds or coulds in your daily habits.

Choose habits that GIVE YOU ENERGY. Most of the daily habits that actually work for people are the ones that add to the person's well being.

"It's more stressful to continue being fat than to stop overeating"

OBSTACLE # 12 Soul Nourishment

We're all scattered for time; kids, spouses, work, family, pets. The list goes on. We're so busy that we rarely make time for the most important person – YOU. It's important for you to just let go - and do something fun for you. When you find that certain "something" that makes you happy – don't let go of it – it's your own personal retreat. This ceremony should be a regular habit for you.

1. No responsibilities required. Choose something that will revive your energy and give you time to forget your daily grind. A walk in the park, drive to the country, stroll a library, warm bath, etc....

2. You're off the clock. This set period of time – is for you only- NO ONE gets this space. You have created this mini-retreat – for only YOU.

3. Pencil ME in. You schedule other important events in your life –DO the same for this ME time. You're equally important and worth it. If I'm not mistaken, there are loved ones in your life who depend on your energy. Keep it up by giving yourself some time off.

If you feel guilty taking this time for yourself – keep reminding yourself that you will be refreshed, rejuvenated, and reenergized.

Look at your life, your family's lives, and your friend's lives. Do you get the feeling that our lives are moving at super speeds, and that we're constantly trying to control it or change it? When you're at home with the kids or at work and there are deadlines to be met – how much "personal' time do you give yourself? You need time alone – an escape – a ritual that's totally yours. You've kept other commitments in your life – why not keep this ritual that's totally yours? You deserve it –you're just as important as your other priorities.

I asked one of our successful clients -who has kept off 40 pounds, Jodi Beight, mother of a six year old, how she gets in touch with her "interior real estate"- that little piece of land in your head that holds a lot of memories-both good and bad. Jodi said she loves to work in her garden. It brings back great memories when her and her mother use to go in and spade the tomatoes. She said it allows her the time to be silent and warms her heart. Jodi realizes that this "gardening" of her own mind slows down her fast pace life and she automatically feels more peaceful.

This little exercise will help you determine the priorities that are important to you.

<u>What do I need in my life right now…?</u> Here is a list of words that can be used to finish the sentence on what you need. ….. mental, emotional, relationships, spiritual, self, etc. The second part of this exercise will be to identify which of these words that can be met by you alone. Then, recognize the words that will require outside support.

Be kind to yourself and don't always be too harsh to judge. Pay attention to what fields your mind tends to sow on a continual basis. You'll feel healthier if you let everything in your mind come in –filter through and knowing that you're aware of your inner thoughts in a much deeper way. This will help you feel more productive in your busy schedule and be more at peace with your hectic, hurried lifestyle.

OBSTACLE # 13 TOP REASONS WHY PEOPLE DON'T EXERCISE

In my twenty years of helping people with their fitness goals, I've heard plenty of excuses why people don't move more. I'm going to tackle the most common reasons head on and deflect every excuse with a few words.

1. **<u>No time in my busy schedule</u>** –My PLAN requires a minimum of 15 minutes every day. Most people who exercise regularly are as busy as –or even busier than---those who are physically inactive.
   Make fitness a priority. It has to become a part of your regular routine – just like brushing your teeth, showering or eating.

2. **<u>No energy</u>**-EXERCISE will BOOST your energy-not take it away.

3. **<u>Can't afford a gym</u>**- All you need is a pair of shoes, so you can walk. I just want you to be more physically active –you can choose household chores to keep fit. My exercise DVD will help tone and firm you.

4. **<u>I don't have room in my home for equipment</u>**- Most of us

don't. You don't need to spend money on expensive equipment or need an "exercise" room with my plan. Small hand held weights can do a great job sculpting your body.

5. <u>**The holidays are coming –can't start now-**</u> There will always be "things" that are coming up. Make YOU your biggest priority. You have the ways that enable you to make your weight management program fit into every daily activity and event in your life.

6. <u>**I travel and most of the hotels don't have gyms-**</u> You can go for walks and see the city you're visiting. Make it a point to bring your walking shoes.

7. <u>**It hurts**</u>- Train don't strain. If it hurts –STOP! Listen to your body. Remember, you don't have to torture your body –for your body to respond favorably.

8. <u>**I have too many pressures in my life right now-**</u> You don't consider eating, showering or brushing your teeth as pressure because they're a part of your regular routine of taking care of yourself. Fitness is another part of your self-care routine – and it has wonderful fringe benefits!

9. <u>**I can't do it alone-**</u> Don't try. Involve people close to you and ask for their encouragement. Find a fitness friend who'll work out with you.

10. <u>**Anxiety over your physical appearance**</u>- Nobody's perfect. We're all individuals. You are unique. You don't look exactly like anyone else – and YOU'RE NOT SUPPOSED to. It's difficult –but try not to compare yourself with any one else.

I know there are more excuses that you can think of, but I can tell you that everyone one of us has the capability of moving more in our lives. Making up excuses solves nothing.

OBSTACLE # 14 WHAT DO I DO ??

A common problem is what to do in certain eating situations. These are a few helpful hints when you're trying to enjoy a meal and still stay within your caloric budget.

WHAT DO I DO …. When I'M HUNGRY BEFORE I GO TO THE RESTAURANT ?
I would advise that you don't leave the house hungry. I believe that ravenous feeling of hunger usually sets you up for a calorie disaster. If I'm hungry and I know I'm going to a restaurant, I usually have an apple or a few nuts to hold me over to avoid pre-meal munching later. This will SAVE you calories in the long run.

WHAT DO I DO….. WHEN I SIT DOWN AT THE TABLE?
It seems like our senses are elevated at this moment. You smell the food, you see the food on other tables–your stomach begins to call your name. This time is important for you to make a good decision. The server will usually ask if you want an appetizer. This is where your temptations and questions start to fire off. Do you or don't you? How hungry are you? If you order an appetizer, can you split it with someone else or is this for you alone? Do I order a decadent choice or a healthy one?

All these questions pop into your head. Split decisions. You can relax. It's perfectly fine to order an appetizer before the meal. You have many healthy options.

- A glass of spicy tomato juice or vegetable drink

- Have one piece of bread with a thin slather of butter

- If you're in a group and they order a fried appetizer platter- just peel off the batter. Remember, most of the fat is in the coating

- Soups are an excellent choice for an appetizer. Bean soups or pea soups are high in fiber and filling, which curbs your hunger. I'd rather you fill up on a split pea soup and salad, than choking down those soggy French fries at the end of your meal because you're still hungry

- Broth-based soups, like minestrone, wonton, beef barley, gazpacho, consommé, or vegetable soup are also wonderful starters to a meal. Avoid the creamy based soups like chowder or bisque, which are loaded with fat and calories

WHAT DO I DO……. AT A SALAD BAR?

A salad bar can be a dieter's nirvana or a place of torment, depending on your discipline, dedication and determination towards your new healthy lifestyle.

I always stick with the staples when I eat at these types of places. I always start off with lettuce and of course, the greener the better. That's when I load up with peppers, cucumbers, carrots, tomatoes, snap peas, raisins, nuts, garbanzo beans, fruit and other fresh produce. I'll even throw in a few eggs with the yolk (that I will discard at my table) that's a heckuva meal in itself.

Want to save some calories-overlook the macaroni salad, croutons, deviled eggs, grated cheeses, creamy dressings, bacon, pasta salad and potato salad.

Lest I remind you, eating "just a little" of 12 different foods turns into "a lot" of food………….calories count!

WHAT DO I DO……….WHEN ORDERING SIDE DISHES?

If you're like most people, you usually think of side dishes as "non-events." They're really not your main course, so it's as if their calories don't count. Think again. These "extras" may be the difference in you gaining or losing. Let's make the smart choices.

Order as many vegetable options as possible. Steamed, stewed or boiled vegetables are best, with little or no added butter or oil. Potato options are good too. Stick with baked, boiled or roasted potatoes. If they only have French fries or chips-ask for a salad in exchange. I always ask for fruit as a side dish. I'll also order just plain rice or pasta with marinara sauce on the side. This choice is better than anything fried or varnished in creamy sauce or gravy.

Avoid anything with butter and cheese sauces. Keep a close eye on anything that has the word 'cream' in it. I guarantee it will not be low in fat.

If you order a baked potato, you can top it off with salsa, lemon juice and pepper, non-fat plain yogurt, steak sauce, low-fat sour cream, or broccoli. I've been known to put barbecue sauce on my baked potato. Hey, don't knock it until you've tried it. If you load up with butter, sour cream, cheese, and bacon bits, you're adding hundreds of calories to your meal.

WHAT DO I DO.......... WHEN ORDERING DESSERTS?

This is the fourth quarter, the ninth inning, the 18 th hole, the last lap–this is the time when superstar athletes put their game face on and this separates the greats from the average ballplayers. You're doing great so far–this is where you can write your legacy to a new healthy lifestyle! You can have a delicious victory at the end of your meals without destroying your daily calorie intake.

OF COURSE, IF YOU'RE FULL - YOU DON'T NEED A DESSERT ....DO YOU? .... DO YOU REALLY??

I 'll always choose fresh fruit as a dessert. However, if it's not available, there's always Sorbet or frozen yogurt. These are great alternatives to ice cream –which is very high in fat. If ice cream is your only choice-keep it to one scoop. Meringue pies are healthier choices. Pumpkin pie is a good choice if you eat the topping and leave the crust. It's not a crime to try a piece of dessert-you don't have to finish the whole piece.

When dining out, make it an automatic with your friends and family-order only one dessert and share it. This satisfies your sweet tooth without packing on the pounds. Mangia!!!

GET LEAN IN 15 will work for YOU as well.............

The Video that Started the Abs Craze!

"After reading through the comments for this video, I have to agree that this is the best ab workout I have found. I played sports throughout high school and college, but now that I've graduated, I find myself going to the gym less often. This video has helped put me back on my fitness schedule and I use it as motivation to get back into the gym. The video does go by fast and I'm already beginning to see the definition in my stomach come back again. If you're looking for a quick, effective program for your stomach, I couldn't recommend anything else."

"I give this short video a ton of credit. It was the perfect choice to kick off a fitness habit five years ago when my girlfriend introduced me to it: the right length to do every day, serious enough to produce results and campy enough to keep me in good humor. It's become an old, reliable friend. In order to keep it handy in my travels, I digitized the videotape so I could play it from my laptop -- then I extracted the audio so I could play it on my iPod! I'll probably still be playing it twenty years from now."

"This tape is what I used to get a flat tummy! For the first time I was so excited to go try on bathing suits in the Summer. It worked wonders as long as you listen to the host and do it exactly how they tell you, don't give up! It works".

"Ever since I bought the :08 minute collection, it has been my favorite workout routine. The videos are very upbeat and focused. And I can look forward to them because I know they're only 8 minutes long. After trying many other video workouts where I could barely keep up, these were a pleasant surprise. **Jaime Brenkus has the right idea by keeping the workouts short and concentrated."**
Customer in Oceanside, CA

I bought the 8-minute abs video about two years ago! **I just recently started using this product and I've lost over 10 pound off my belly and 5 on my not so loveable love handles! This video really works I recommend this video to anyone who's serious about their body!!!**
Ashlee of Florida

I began using 8 Minute Abs over five years ago when the video was relatively new. **I had a 34-inch waist. After one month of doing the video every morning faithfully, I had trimmed my waist to an incredible 32 inches without a change in diet. My mother, who had a 44-inch waist, noticed the change on me and began doing the video with me. She lost around 4 inches on her waist after about six weeks.** I am even more impressed now. **I have what many would call "perfect abs" and I owe all of my thanks to this video**. My only criticism, if you can call it that, is that the front of the stomach becomes flatter quicker than the "love handle" area.
James of Kansas

I have been working out for several years now and not really getting any results from setups. I tried the tape and kept going'. **After a week I noticed a difference. I went from a 38" waist to a 36".** The main thing is that it keeps you going without getting boring. 9 Exercises for 45 seconds and you hit all the moves. First thing in the morning I hit the tape and after 8 short minutes it's over and you get results. **It's great having a personal trainer in your living room everyday and getting results.**
John of California

Before   After

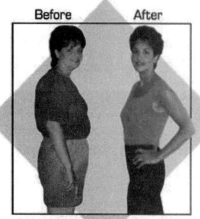

Sandy Bihlmeyer, Lost 25 pounds.
Size 12 to size 6.

Before   After

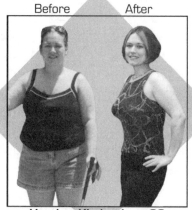

Heather Kinder, Lost 60
pounds, went down from size
20 to size 9

Before   After

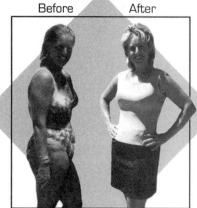

Shari Palumbo, Lost 37 pounds

Before   After

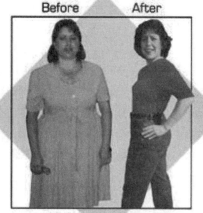

Jodi Beight, Lost 40 pounds.
Dropped 4 pant sizes.

Before   After

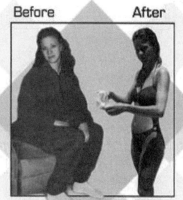

Pam Sluga, Lost 28 pounds.
Dropped 4 pant sizes.

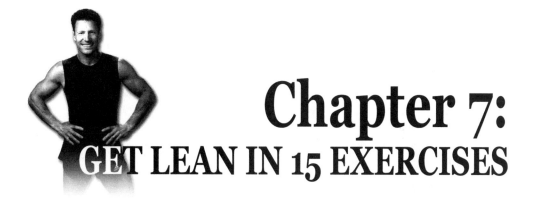

Chapter 7:
GET LEAN IN 15 EXERCISES

The following photos will show you exactly how to do each exercise with perfect form. You were given my 15 Day exercise plan in Chapter 4. However, if you would like to mix and match, I have devised a special 15 minute workout plan for you utilizing this Chapter;

Choose 5 exercises from the **UPPER BODY** section
Choose 5 exercises from the **LOWER BODY** section
Choose 5 exercises from the **ABS & BUNS** section
  • Do each exercise for **10-15** repetitions
  • Do each exercise **2X (twice)**
  • Enjoy looking at your new body !

UPPER
1. Push ups
2. Chest Press
3. Chest Flys
4. Standing Rows
5. One Arm Rows
6. Shoulder Press
7. Lateral Raises
8. Front Raises
9. Rear Shoulder Raises
10. Bicep Curls
11. Concentrated Curls
12. Triceps Kickback
13. Triceps Press
14. Dips on Chair

LOWER
1. Squats
2. Plie Squats
3. One Leg Squats
4. Stationary Lunges
5. Alternating Lunges
6. Reverse Lunges
7. Straight Leg Dead Lifts
8. Quad Lifts
9. Outer Thigh Lifts
10. Frog Kicks
11. Inner Thigh Lifts

ABS & BUNS

ABS
1. Crunches
2. Side Crunches
3. Reverse Crunches
4. Bicycles
5. Scrunches
6. Overhead Crunches

BUNS
1. Buns Press
2. Buns Kicks
3. Buns Lifts
4. Standing Buns Press

Modified Push Ups	Please follow these guidelines: Modified Push Ups. Begin in a modified push up position. You will be on your hands and knees as opposed to extending your legs. Make sure your hands are a bit wider than your shoulders. Slowly lower yourself -about three or four inches from the floor. Your elbows should be bent at 90 degrees. Keep your abs tight and your back straight throughout the movement, and gently push yourself up without locking the elbows. This exercise firms the chest, shoulders and back of the arms. *Do each rep with a 3 second count

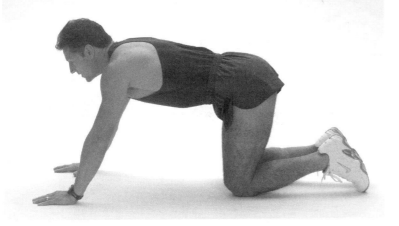

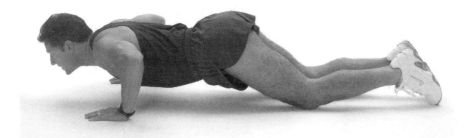

| **Chest Press** | Please follow these guidelines: Chest Press. Lying down on your back with your knees bent at 90 degrees. Place hand-held weights a few inches above your chest and slowly push your arms upward. Keep the weights a few inches apart and make sure that you don't lock out the elbows. Control the movement down to your chest. This firms the chest muscles.
*Do each rep with a 3 second count |

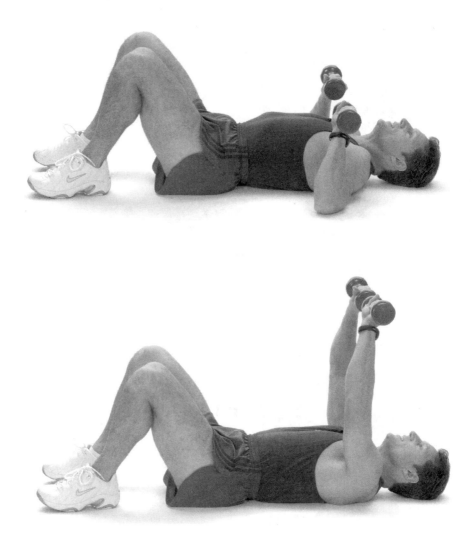

Chest Flys	Please follow these guidelines: Chest Flys. Lying down on your back. Keep your knees bent at 90 degrees and feet flat on the floor. Press hand-held weights up over your chest with the palms facing each other. Now, move your arms in an arc motion–like you're "hugging a barrel." Slowly lower your arms to the starting position and repeat. Flys concentrate on your outer chest muscles and helps firm and tone the entire chest. *Do each rep with a 3 second count

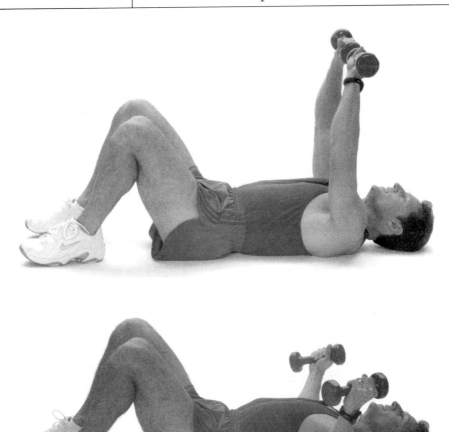

Standing Rows	Please follow these guidelines: Standing Rows. Standing with small hand-held weights in front of your thighs. Slightly bend at the waist while keeping your knees bent and your back straight. Slowly pull the weights back like you were rowing a boat. Pull your shoulders back and keep your chest out. Try not to lean back. This is a steady, controlled movement. This firms up the "bra strap" line and the back muscles. *Do each rep with a 3 second count

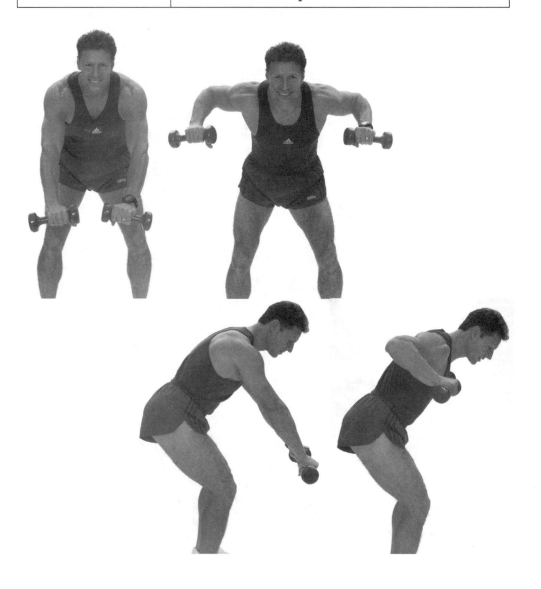

One Arm Rows	Please follow these guidelines: One Arm Rows: Place one of your knees on a chair and support your body with your hand on the chair. Lean forward bending at your waist and let the weight hang at your side about shin level. Slowly pull the weight up by following the contour of your body – don't twist your body. Keep your abs tight. Focus on pulling with your back – like you're starting a lawnmower. This exercise creates that tapered "v" look. – Building your back muscles – makes your waist look smaller. *Do each rep with a 3 second count

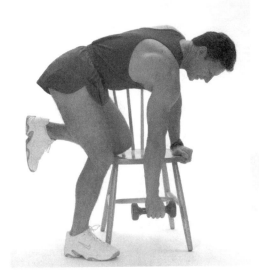

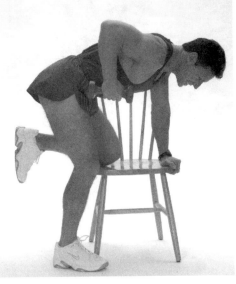

| **Shoulder Press** | Please follow these guidelines: Shoulder Press. Slightly bend your knees, while keeping your abs tight and back straight. Hold two hand-held weights or any resistance you have in the home (soup cans, milk jugs, tubing , etc...) just above your shoulder level. Keep your palms faced out when you hold the resistance. Press the resistance straight up until they're almost touching. This is a slow and controlled movement. Please don't lock out your elbows. This exercise strengthens your entire shoulder muscle.
*Do each rep with a 3 second count |

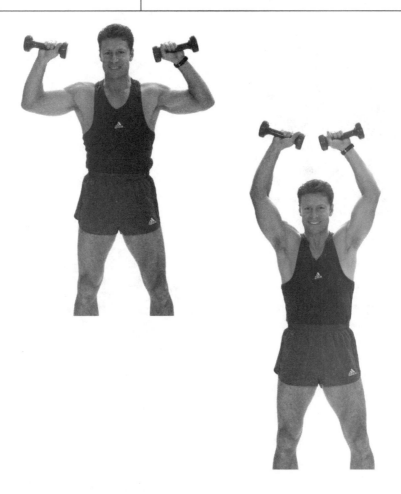

Lateral Raises	Please follow these guidelines: Lateral Raises. Start with the resistance at your side. Slowly raise the resistance out to your sides until they reach shoulder level. Your palms should be faced down, like your pouring tea. Your elbows should be slightly bent throughout this slow and controlled movement. Lateral Raises emphasize the middle portion of your shoulder, which makes your waist look smaller. *Do each rep with a 3 second count

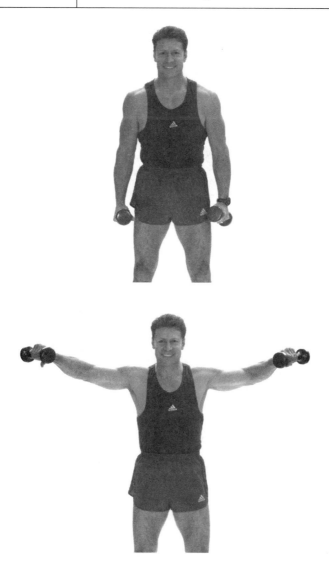

Front Raises	Please follow these guidelines: Front Raises. Standing straight with your knees slightly bent, abs held tight and back straight. Place hand-held weights with an overhand grip in front of your thighs. Slowly raise the weights to eye level and then lower to starting position. Don't swing the weights –stay in control. This helps shape the front shoulder. *Do each rep with a 3 second count

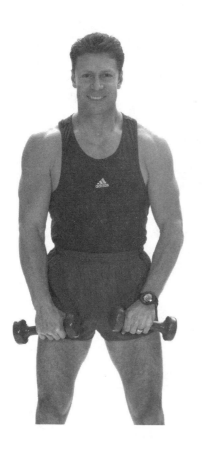
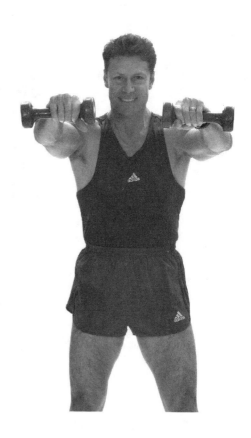

Rear Shoulder Raises	Please follow these guidelines: Rear Shoulder Raises. Bending at the waist, keeping your knees bent, abs tight and back straight. Place hand-held weights in front of you with the palms faced inward. Slowly raise the weights out to your sides with your elbows slightly bent. At the highest point in the movement – squeeze your shoulder blades together and slowly lower. This concentrates on the back portion of the shoulder muscle. *Do each rep with a 3 second count

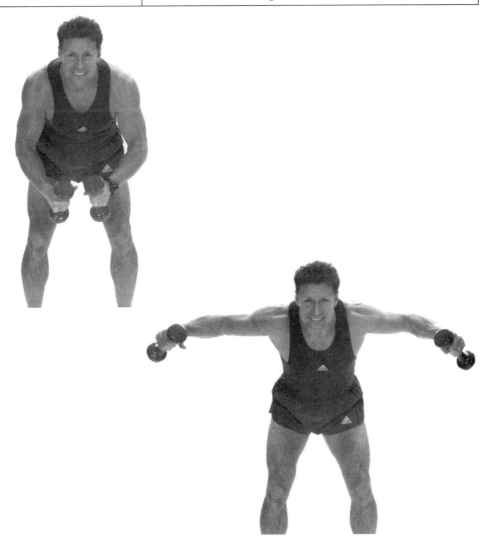

Bicep Curls	Please follow these guidelines: Bicep Curls. Stand with your knees slightly bent, abs tight, and keep your back straight. Your feet should be hip-width apart. Hold the hand-held weights on the outside of your thighs. Slowly curl the weights up toward your shoulders. Keep nice controlled movement --don't swing the arms ! This focuses on the front of your arms. *Do each rep with a 3 second count

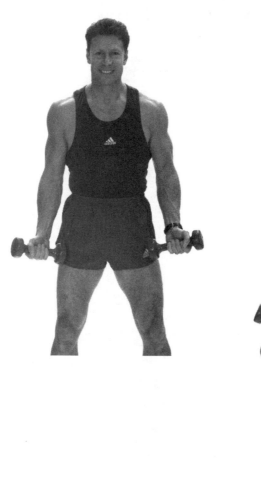
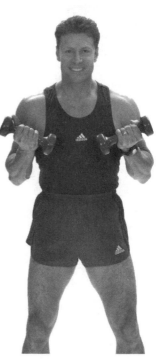

Concentration Curls	Please follow these guidelines: Concentration Curls. Sitting on a chair or you can do this exercise kneeling on the floor. Place your elbow on your inner thigh and lean into the leg to raise your elbow for proper range of motion. Curl the weight up to the front of your shoulder –squeezing the muscle at the top peak of the exercise. Don't forget to alternate sides. This really isolates the bicep muscle. *Do each rep with a 3 second count

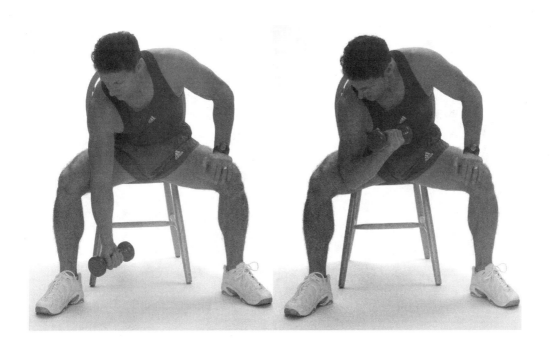

Triceps Kickbacks	Please follow these guidelines: Triceps Kickbacks. Stand in a split stance with a small hand-held weight. Bend forward at your waist and put your opposite hand on your knee for added support. Bring the weight up by keeping your elbow next to your torso. Slowly straighten the arm out and make sure that you don't lock out the elbow joint. The KEY is to keep your elbow up for a full range of motion. Slow and steady movements. This exercise tightens and firms up the back of the arms. *Do each rep with a 3 second count

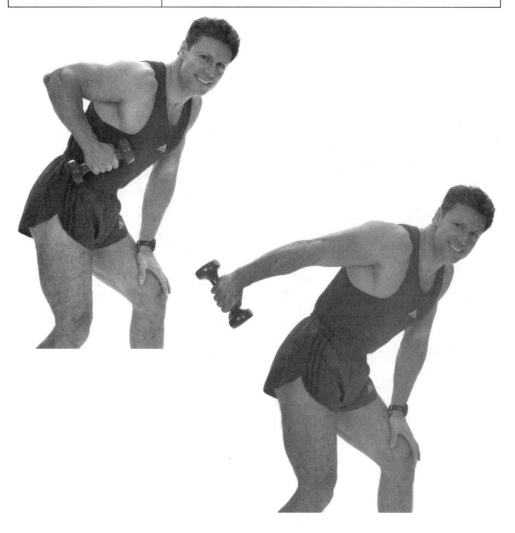

Triceps Press	Please follow these guidelines: Triceps Press. Standing straight with your knees slightly bent and your abs held tight. Clasp both weights in your hands and extend your arms overhead. Keep your elbows close to your ears and slowly lower weights behind you – until your elbows are at 90 degrees. Beware--don't clunk yourself in the head on this movement. This tones and firms that "wiggly, jiggly" back of the arm muscle. *Do each rep with a 3 second count

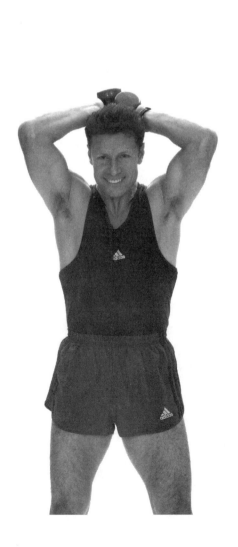
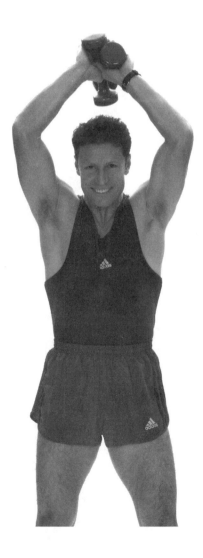

Dips on Chair	Please follow these guidelines: Dips on Chair. Sitting on a chair, placing your hands next to your hips. Lift your hips off the chair and slowly lower your body until your elbows are at 90 degrees and then lift yourself back up. Keep your knees bent throughout the movement. However, if you're advanced – you can straighten your legs. Keep your body close to the chair when you're lowering it. These dips tone and firm the back of the arms -your triceps. *Do each rep with a 3 second count

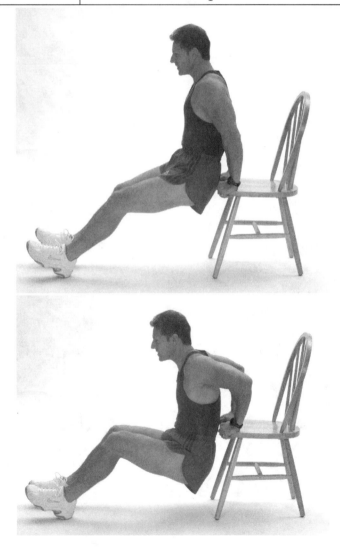

Squats	Please follow these guidelines: Squats. Your feet should be shoulder width apart. Your abs are held in tight and your back is straight. Place your hands out in front about chest level. Slowly lower yourself into a seating position- until you touch your buns on the seat. Make sure your knees don't go past your toes and are aligned straight. Do this exercise with controlled, slow movements. **If you want more of a challenge, you can also use hand held weights at your sides while doing this exercise. This is the single best leg shaper. It tones your buns, thighs, hamstrings and quads. *Do each rep with a 3 second count

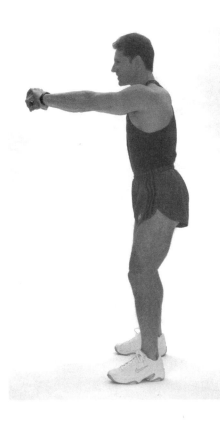
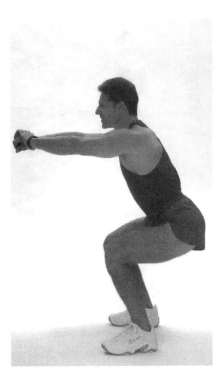

Plie Squats	Please follow these guidelines: Plie Squats. Standing up, place your feet in the 10 o'clock and 2 o'clock position. Slowly lower your body into a squat position -stick those buns out – like you're sitting in a seat. Keep your knees in line with your toes. Keep your abs tight and your back straight. If you want added resistance – hold hand-held weights at your side. This really shapes your entire lower body with emphasis on the inner thighs. *Do each rep with a 3 second count

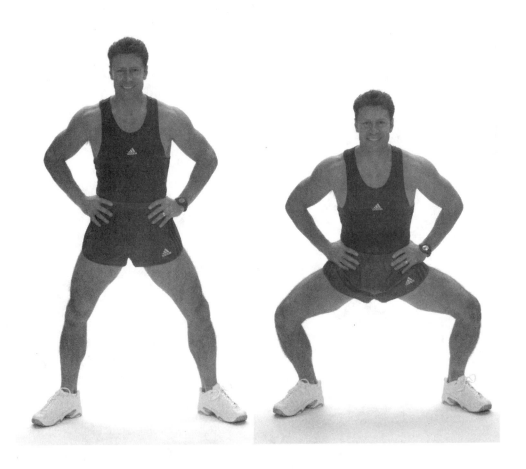

One Leg Squats	Please follow these guidelines: One Leg Squats. Standing up straight on one leg. Bend your opposite leg 90 degrees. Slowly tip forward from your hips and lower your torso towards the floor and raise yourself back up. Keep your abs tight and back flat throughout this movement. Squeeze your buns and tighten up the back of the leg as you do this exercise. This firms your hamstring muscles- the back of your legs and your buns. 　　　*Do each rep with a 3 second count

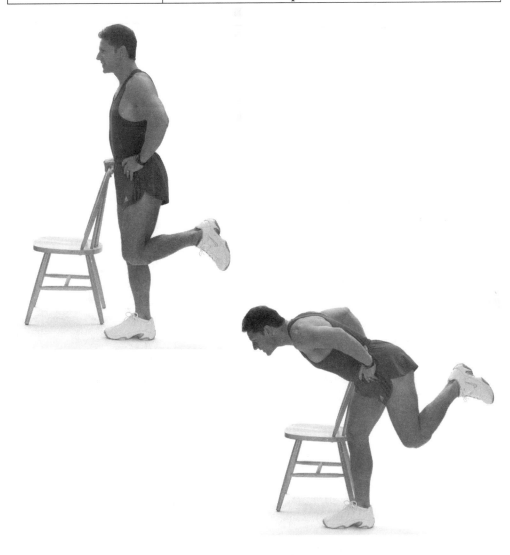

Stationary Lunges	Please follow these guidelines: Stationary Lunges. You should use a chair for balance and support. Stand in a split stance with you feet about three feet apart –the wider the better. Slowly lower your body down until your front knee is bent at 90 degrees and your back knee is bent towards the floor. The KEY to this movement is to make sure your front knee stays behind the toes and is aligned straight. Keep your abs tight and your back straight. As you progress, you can hold a small hand-held weight at your side. This exercise strengthens and firms your buns, hamstrings, front thighs and hips. *Do each rep with a 3 second count

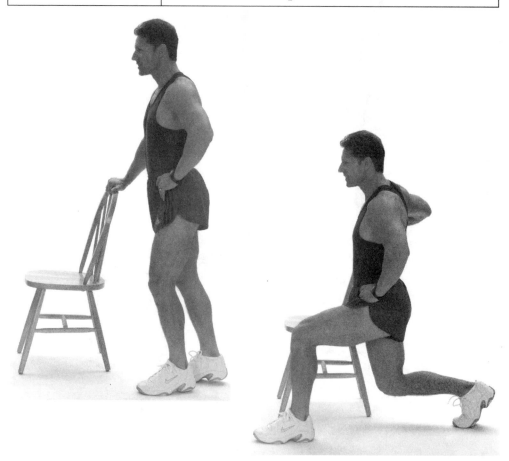

Alternating Lunges	Please follow these guidelines: Alternating Lunges. Standing with your feet together – slowly step with right foot forward into a lunge movement. Don't allow your front knee to go past the toes and keep the knee aligned with your toes. Always keep your abs tight –and back straight. Alternate legs by lunging forward with your left foot – continue alternating legs. Think of this movement like a "fencer" in the Olympics. This trains the entire lower body; hips, buns, quads and hamstrings. *Do each rep with a 3 second count

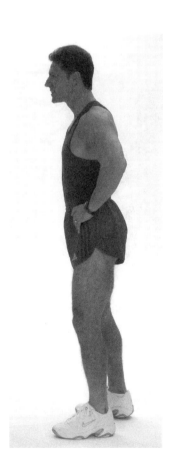
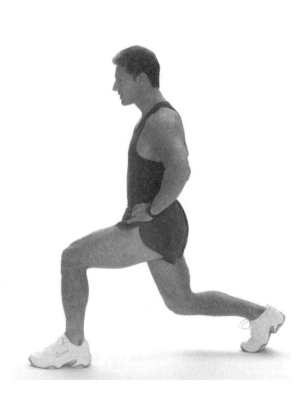

Reverse Lunges	Please follow these guidelines: Reverse Lunges. I recommend using a chair for balance and support. Stand with your feet together. Slowly step back about 3 feet. Bend both of your knees – and lower yourself in a controlled movement. Don't allow your front knee to bend over your toe. Don't push with the back foot – use your front leg to pull your back leg in. As always, keep your abs tight and back straight. This exercise is a great overall lower body shaper.
	*Do each rep with a 3 second count

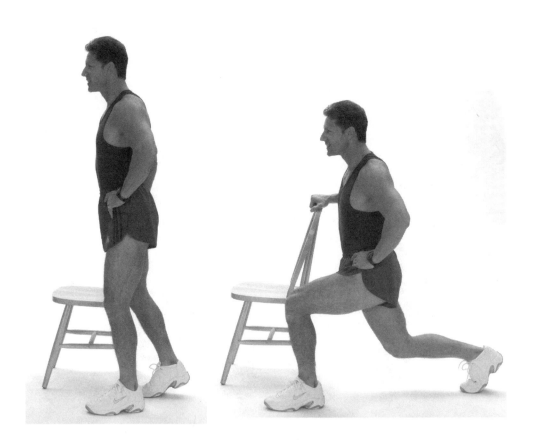

Straight Leg Dead Lifts	Please follow these guidelines: Straight Leg Dead Lifts. Stand with your feet hip-width apart. Rest hand-held weights on your front thighs. Slowly tip over from your hips and lower your body as far as your flexibility allows. Slowly raise up. Keep your back straight and abs tight. *Don't round your back. Squeeze your buns to get the maximum effect! Great for your buns, back of your legs and lower back. *Do each rep with a 3 second count

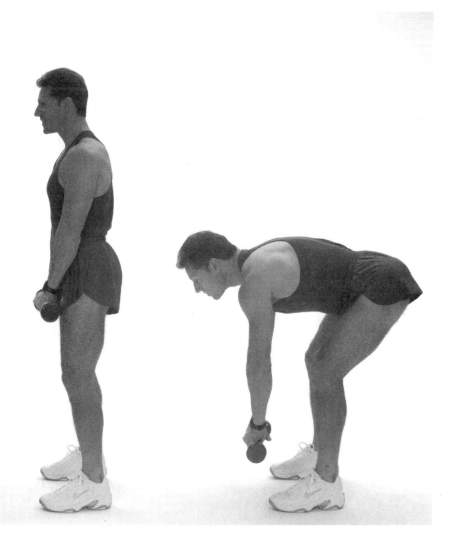

Quad Lifts	Please follow these guidelines: Quad Lifts. Lie on the floor on your back. Keep one knees bent at 90 degrees and straighten your opposite leg and lift it up until perpendicular to floor (or as high as you can). Slowly lower your leg back to the starting position. Tighten your abs to keep your back from arching. Switch legs after appropriate reps. This Lift targets your quads-the front of your thighs and hip flexors If you want too progress, you can add light ankle weights. 　　　　*Do each rep with a 3 second count

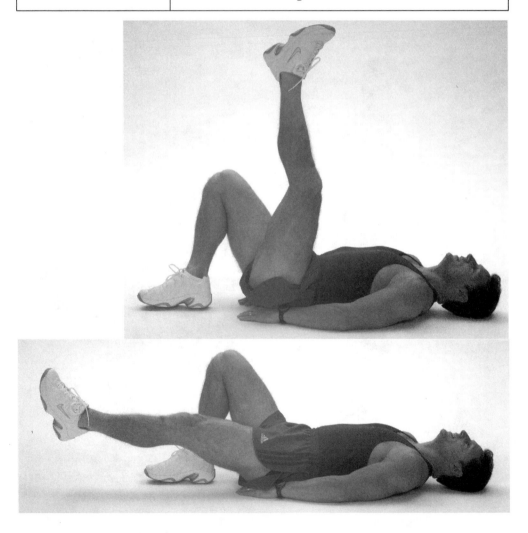

Outer Thigh Lifts	Please follow these guidelines: Outer Thigh Lifts. You'll need a chair for balance and support. Standing up straight, bend one knee at 90 degrees and slowly lift your bent leg straight out and lower. Always keep the knee bent during this movement. You don't have to go up too high. Keep you abs tight and your back straight. Try not to lean during the movement. For added resistance, you can use ankle weights or place your hand on your outer thigh area and monitor the resistance. As always, slow and controlled movements. This exercise concentrates on the "saddle bag" area. *Do each rep with a 3 second count

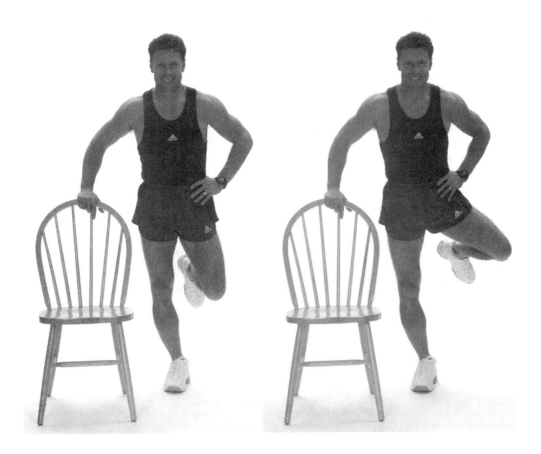

Frog Kicks	Please follow these guidelines: Frog Kicks. Lying on your back on the floor placing your hands under your buns. Bend both of your knees at 90 degrees. Lift your legs in the 10 o' clock and 2 o' clock position and kick your legs out at a 45 degree angle. This is a slow and controlled movement. For added resistance, use ankle weights. *Do each rep with a 3 second count

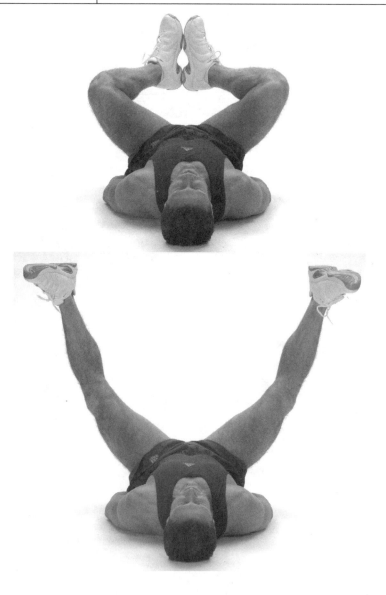

Inner Thigh Lifts	Please follow these guidelines: Inner Thigh Lifts. Lying down on your side–support your body with your arm. Keep your top leg bent and straighten out your bottom leg. Flex your foot and slowly lift the leg up. You don't have to lift too high. Keep your movements steady and slow. For added intensity you can place small weights on your inner thigh, use ankle weights or place one hand on the moving leg and monitor the resistance yourself. Switch sides after you finish the appropriate reps. This exercise targets your inner thigh area. *Do each rep with a 3 second count

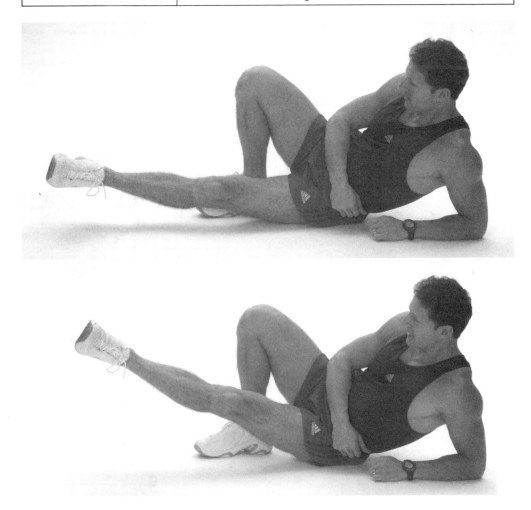

Crunches	Please follow these guidelines: Crunches. Lie on your back on the floor with your knees bent at 90 degrees. Place your hands just behind your ears–this will ensure that you don't pull on your neck. Look up towards the ceiling and imagine an orange placed between your chin and chest-so your head stays nice and straight. Slowly lift your shoulders off the floor-you don't have to go up too high. You will feel your abdominal muscles contracting as you lift up. Do these movements slow and controlled. Gives you a slimmer, trimmer, tighter waistline. *Do each rep with a 3 second count

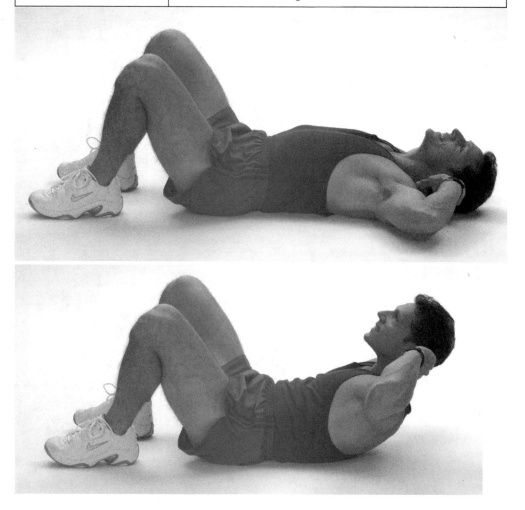

Side Crunches	Please follow these guidelines: Side Crunches. Lying down on your back. Keep your knees bent at 90 degrees and gently shift them over to one side. Place one hand behind your ear. Slowly lift your shoulders off the floor. Again, reminding you that you should not yank on your neck do your assigned reps on one side and then switch. This exercise work's the "love handles." *Do each rep with a 3 second count

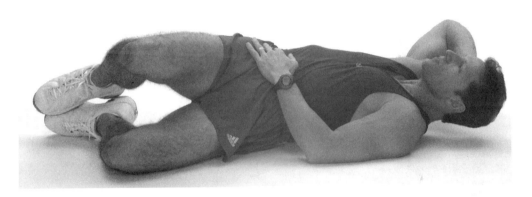

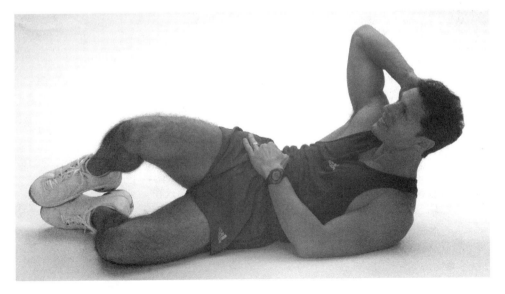

| **Reverse Crunches** | Please follow these guidelines: Reverse Crunches. Lie on the floor on your back and place your hands under your buns. Keep your knees bent at 90 degrees and slowly curl your hips off the floor and bring them towards your chest. You can keep your feet together or cross them during this movement. This is a small move, so don't rock and create momentum –keep it slow and steady. This firms the lower region of the abs.

*Do each rep with a 3 second count |

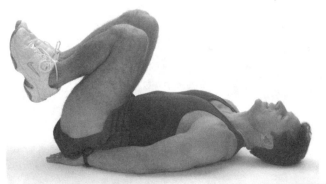

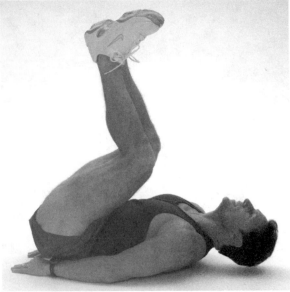

Bicycles	Please follow these guidelines: Bicycles. Lying down on your back–your knees are up and bent at 90 degrees. Place your fingers behind your ears-don't pull on your neck. Slowly bring your knees into your chest –alternating each leg to opposite elbow –in a pedaling motion. Your right elbow goes to your left knee and left elbow to the right knee. Keep switching sides-don't bring the legs out to far –this puts stress on your lower back. Bicycles focus on the entire abdominal region with an emphasis on the obliques (love handles). *Do each rep with a 3 second count

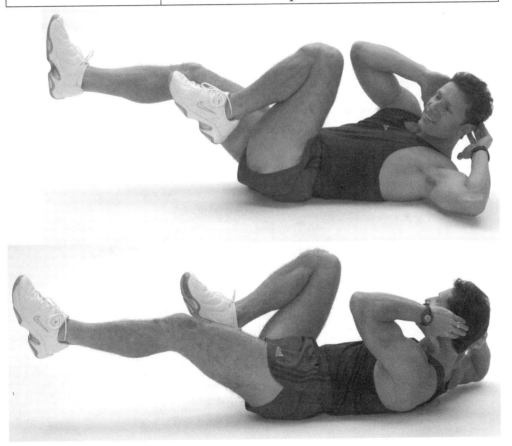

Scrunches	Please follow these guidelines: Scrunches. Lying down on your back on the floor. Keep your knees bent at 90 degrees- place fingers behind your ears. Curl your knees up to the chest –while doing a basic crunch. Bring your feet back down to the floor and repeat. This is a small controlled movement -don't arch your back to gain momentum. This targets the entire ab area. *Do each rep with a 3 second count

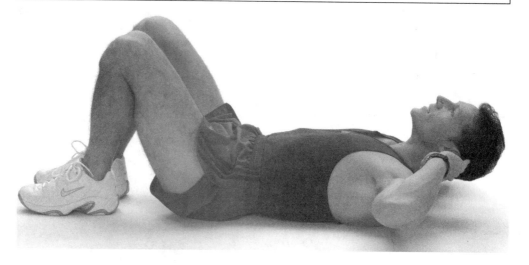

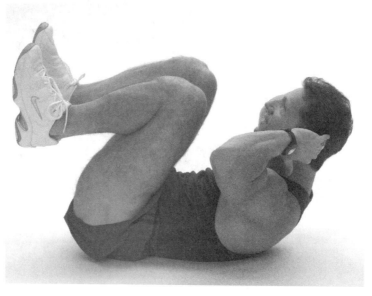

| **Overhead Crunches** | Please follow these guidelines: Overhead Crunches. Lying on your back on the floor –your knees are bent at 90 degrees. Extend your arms overhead – while you slowly curl your body up –like a basic Crunch.

Just lift your shoulders off the ground 30 degrees. Slowly lower and repeat. This advanced Crunch will tighten your abs in no time.

*Do each rep with a 3 second count |

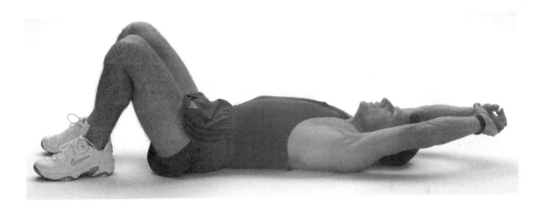

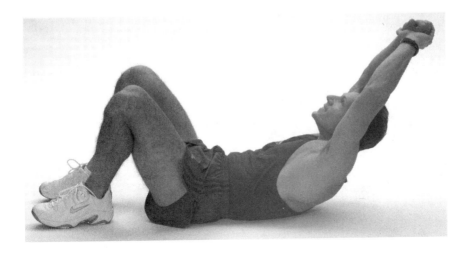

Buns Press	Please follow these guidelines: Buns Press. Position yourself on the floor on your elbows and knees. Bend your knee, flex your foot and keep it at 90 degrees throughout the movement. Keep lifting your leg -like you're stomping bugs on the ceiling. Don't arch your back-and keep your abs tight. Repeat all reps before switching sides. Add ankle weights for more intensity. Lets burn those buns ! *Do each rep with a 3 second count

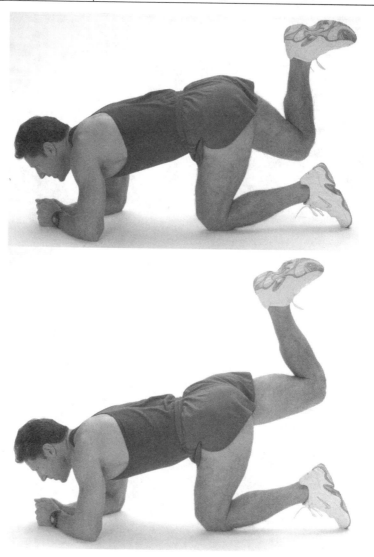

Buns Kicks	Please follow these guidelines: Buns Kicks. You will position yourself on the floor on your elbows and knees. Bring one leg in towards your chest and then slowly extend it outwards. Don't arch your back or bring the leg up too high. Keep your abs tight and your back straight. Do this movement slowly and controlled. Do all your reps before switching legs. You can add ankle weights for more intensity. This exercise will give you a firmer, rounded, uplifted appearance to your buns ! *Do each rep with a 3 second count

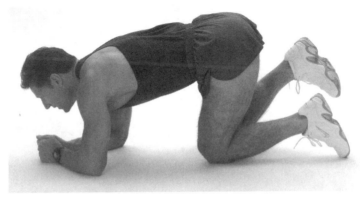

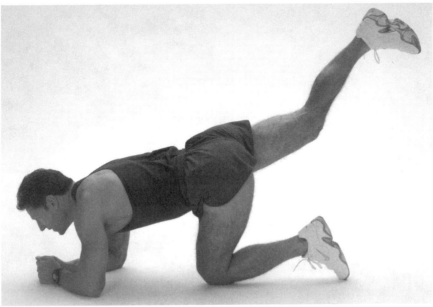

Buns Lifts	Please follow these guidelines: Buns Lifts. You'll position yourself on your elbows and knees on the floor. Extend one leg straight and just lift that leg until it's parallel with the floor. Don't lift up too high-and don't arch your back. Slowly lower and control the movements so your not swinging the leg. For added resistance, you can add ankle weights. These Lifts warm those buns ! *Do each rep with a 3 second count

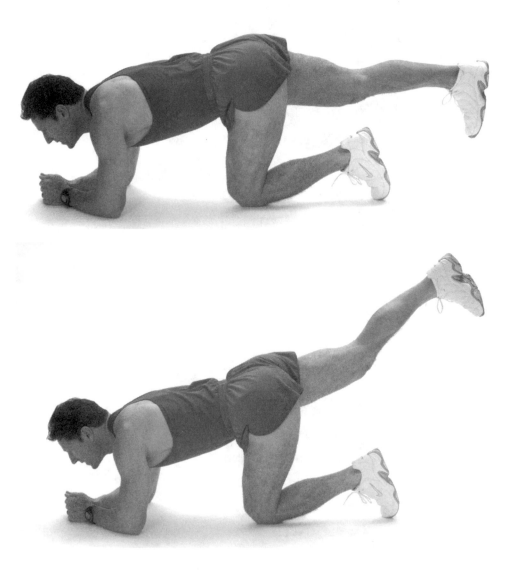

Standing Buns Press (beginners)	Follow these guidelines: Standing Buns Press. If you don't feel comfortable getting on the floor you can do a similar movement standing up. Holding onto a chair for support, bend one leg in a 90 degree position and push back. Keep your back straight and make sure that you don't arch your back. Switch legs after appropriate reps. Focuses on giving you a firmer, rounded uplifted appearance in your buns. *Do each rep with a 3 second count

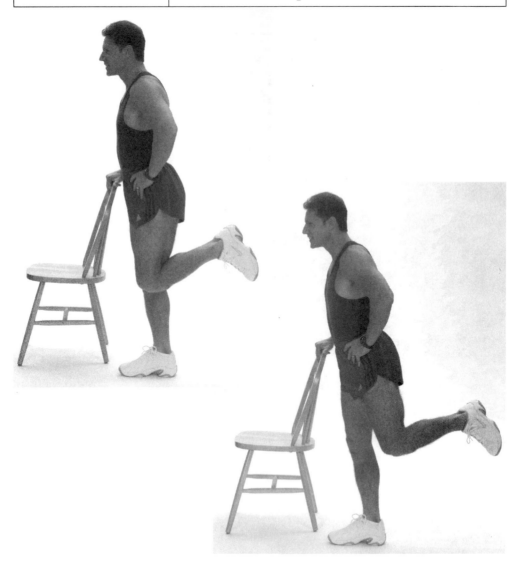

STRETCHES

While you stretch, make sure you breathe and don't bounce through the stretch. When you start feeling the "pull," then that's far enough.

Shoulder Stretch	Stand and extend right arm in front of body. With your left hand located above the right elbow, pull right elbow across chest toward left shoulder. Hold 10 to 15 seconds. Repeat on the other side.

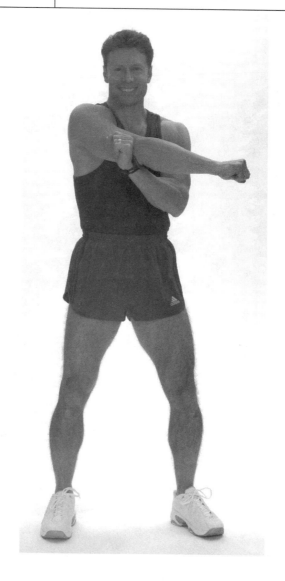

| **Triceps Stretch** | Stand with your arms overhead. Hold your elbow with hand of opposite arm. Gently pull your elbow behind your head. Hold 10 to 15 seconds. Repeat on the other side. |

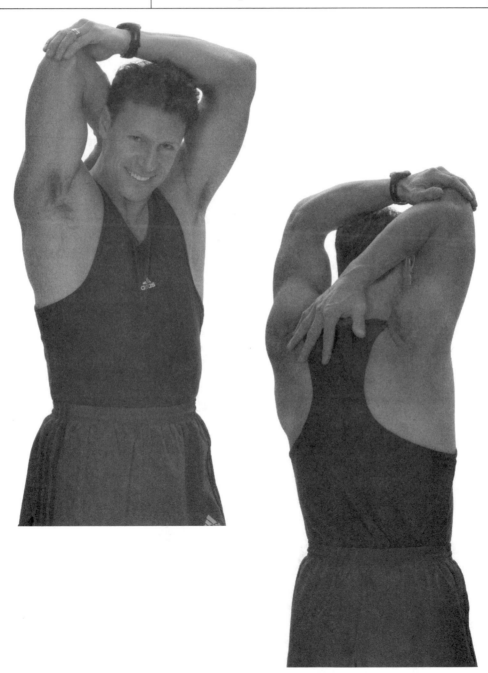

| Quad Stretch | Holding on to a chair. Stand straight, grasp top of left foot with left hand and pull heel towards your buns. Make sure the knees are together. Hold 10 to 15 seconds. Repeat on the other side. |

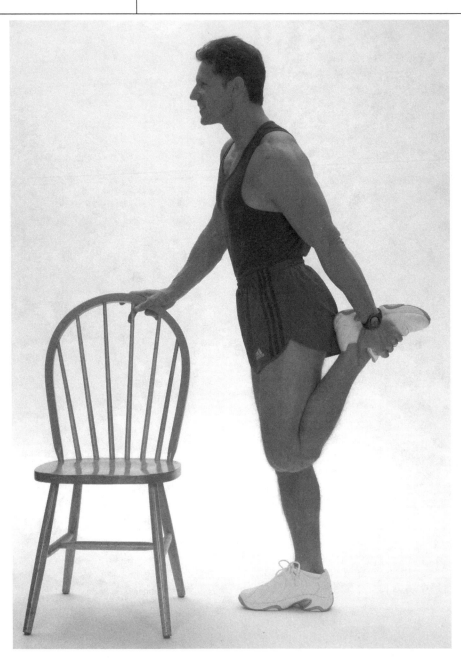

Hamstring Stretch	Sit with one leg straight and your other leg bent. With your back straight and your head up, slowly lean forward at your waist. You should feel the stretch along the underside of your thigh. Hold 10 to 15 seconds. Repeat on the other side.

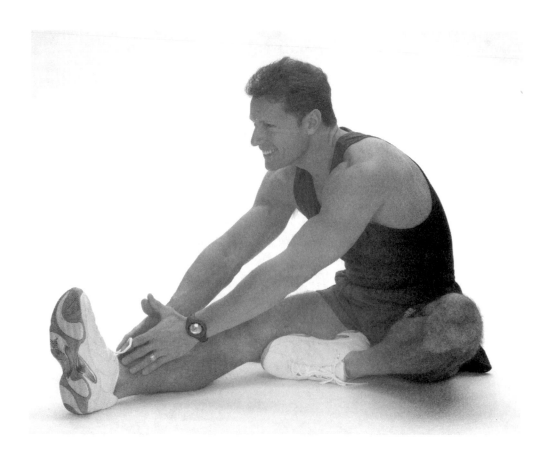

Groin Stretch	Sit with your feet together, your back is straight and your head up. Keep your elbows on the inside of your knees. Then slowly push down on the inside of your knees with your elbows. You should feel the stretch along the inside of your thighs. Hold the stretch for 10 to 15 seconds.

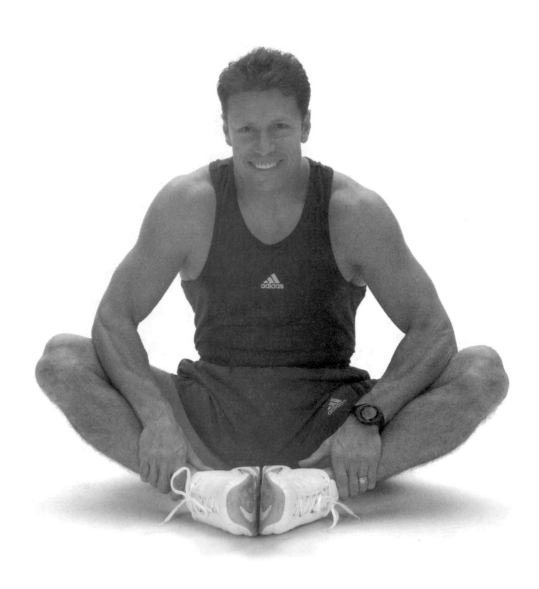

Lower Back Release	Lying on your back, bring both knees into the chest and hold for 10 –15 seconds. Don't rock

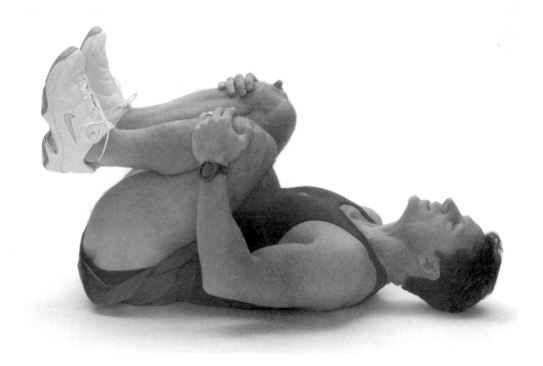

| **Lower Back Stretch** | Lying on your back, keep your shoulders on the ground. Bring one leg across your body by moving only the hips in that direction. Hold for 10-15 seconds and repeat on the other side. |

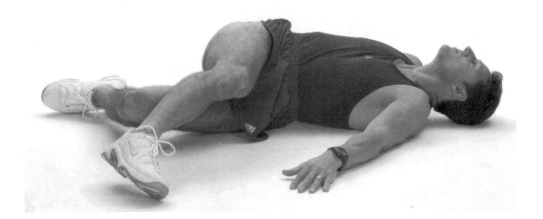

LEARN IT

LIVE IT

LOSE IT...

YOU'LL LOVE IT!!!!

GET LEAN IN 15

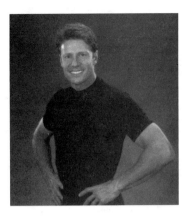

ABOUT THE AUTHOR

Jaime Brenkus is a nationally recognized fitness guru, famous for his ability to take simple, tried-and-true health concepts and market them as exciting, consumer-friendly innovations. One of his biggest successes is the 8-minute Abs workout video series which has helped millions of people. This series is such a winner, it has become a cultural icon, immortalized in Ben Stiller's blockbuster movie, There's Something About Mary.

Jaime is the lead visionary on a new website called Fit15.com that will teach its members how to become Healthy, Wealthy and Wise.

Brenkus is designing the SLIM-FAST Virtual Fitness Trainer program that will be featured on the Slim-Fast on-line community.

In 2006, Jaime was awarded a partner in the 50th Anniversary of the President's Council on Physical Fitness & Sports. This endeavor celebrates 50 years of physical activity, sports, and fitness and advocates the new slogan, GET AMERICA MOVING!

Jaime designed supermodel Kathy Ireland's exercise video, *Bodyspecifics and Reach*; it was named 1997 health and fitness video of the year by the Video and Software Distributors Association (VSDA). He is the co-designer of the *Perfect Portions Diet Dish* – one of the inspirations for this book – a product that's endorsed by many prominent weight loss scientists and experts. To date, nearly 200,000 dishes have been sold. Among Brenkus's 50 video, infomercial, commercial, spokesperson and home shopping channel TV appearances, he was featured in the *Body By*

Jake "Energize Yourself" fitness video, and appeared with Cher in a Bally's Fitness national commercial.

Jaime is certified by the American College of Sports Medicine (ACSM) and has been nominated for a position on the President's Council on Physical Fitness and Sports.

Jaime's resume features his impressive success as a Personal Trainer in Los Angeles, Tampa and Cleveland with live TV appearances in these markets.

Jaime's highly effective and inspiring presentation of pertinent health and fitness issues springs out of substantial natural style and formal study in obtaining his BA Degree in Communication from the University of South Florida in 1983.

Here's what some of his fans say:

KATHY IRELAND, Supermodel, and Producer of videos on physical fitness: "I'm always looking for new ways to exercise effectively and efficiently, so I turned to an expert in the field. His name is Jaime Brenkus."

Dr. Michael Scher, Tampa, Fl: "Following Jaime's program, I lost 40 pounds. It's the only approach that gave me long-term results. I highly endorse the Low fat N Fit Kit. It really works."

Robert Needham, JD, FranchiseInc!: "Jaime Brenkus is an updated reminder of young Jack Lalanne in his personable, non-radical, common sense, consumer-advocate approach to health and fitness. Jaime's bright personality, commanding presence and down to earth, believable style is quite compelling and very compatible with any marketing position advocating healthy lifestyles. His overall program is an economical, easy to assume, non-dieting lifestyle of body management through smart eating and moderate, fun exercises."

JoAnne Denk, Home Shopping Showcase: "Jaime is compelling, energetic and legitimate. In an overcrowded marketing arena, he is genuinely concerned about helping people improve their bodies and their lives. Jaime is living proof of the success of his program, sporting a tightly contoured body and an upbeat, positive outlook on life. This is a proven successful DRTV product category waiting for its next fitness idol to emerge, and he could be the next Jack Lalane."

Donna Rosen, Cleveland, OH: "I am, without a doubt, a major success story. I used to weigh 317 pounds. Thankfully, just when I thought I had reached the end of my rope, Jaime Brenkus came into my life. I went on his program and within the first month, I lost 20 pounds. Now, a little over a year later, I have lost an amazing 158 pounds. I have gone from a dress size 28 to 16. If I can do it, I know you can too!"

Ben J. Meola, R.N., M.S.: "The benefits of Jaime's program are well documented. The positive modifications you make today will be well worth the effort tomorrow."